STRENGTH TRAINING FOR WOMEN

JOHN SHEPHERD

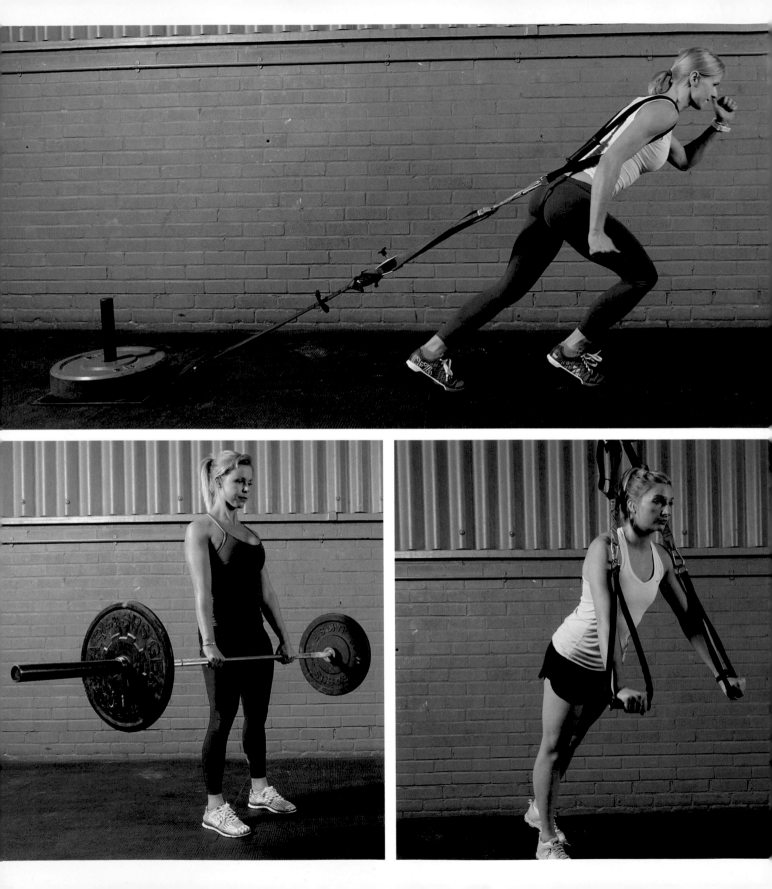

BLOOMSBURY

STRENGTH TRAINING FOR WOMEN

JOHN SHEPHERD

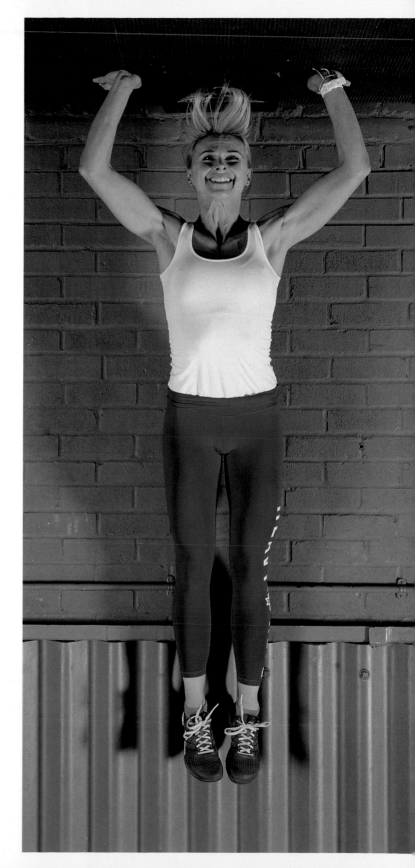

Bloomsbury Sport

An imprint of Bloomsbury Publishing Plc

50 Bedford Square	1385 Broadway
London	New York
WC1B 3DP	NY 10018
UK	USA

www.bloomsbury.com

BLOOMSBURY and the Diana logo are trademarks of Bloomsbury Publishing Plc

First published in 2016

British Library Cataloguing-in-Publication Data

A catalogue record for this book is available from the British Library.

Library of Congress Cataloguing-in-Publication data has been applied for.

ISBN: PB 978-1-4729-1719-5

ePDF: 978-1-4729-1721-8

ePub: 978-1-4729-1720-1

2 4 6 8 10 9 7 5 3 1

Typeset in Nimbus Sans Novus T by Sunrise Studios

Printed and bound in China by C&C Offset Printing Co., Ltd

Bloomsbury Publishing Plc makes every effort to ensure that the papers used in the manufacture of our books are natural, recyclable products made from wood grown in well-managed forests. Our manufacturing processes conform to the environmental regulations of the country of origin.

To find out more about our authors and books visit www.bloomsbury.com. Here you will find extracts, author interviews, details of forthcoming events and the option to sign up for our newsletters.

Contents

1 WHY *WEIGHT*? YOUR JOURNEY TO A NEW YOU STARTS NOW!

Welcome to *Strength Training for Women*. I'm John Shepherd and I've been writing on health, nutrition and sports and fitness training for over 20 years. In this time I've also trained a lot of people from all backgrounds and levels of fitness and abilities and for numerous purposes and goals. I wanted to write this book to explain why resistance training (training against your body weight, with a suspension trainer or with added weight, such as kettlebells or barbells) is so important for women. In my many years in fitness and sport I've heard many negative comments, opinions and falsities on the subject of women and resistance training, so it's my aim to put these to bed and to encourage women to resistance train. I believe it could be the single most important decision you'll ever make regarding how you work out. And it could benefit you in so many other aspects of your life, too. Many women who train the 'resistance way' experience a boost in confidence and feel better just going about their daily lives.

In what I refer to as the 'gymscape', i.e. the world of gyms, there can appear be an order to things when it comes to working out and selecting training options. It's a sort of gender-divide, and is relevant to the subject matter of this book. Men are naturally drawn to lifting weights – and often initially unrealistic ones at that! – while women tend to go for more 'creative' fitness options such as dance-based classes, like Zumba® or one of the multitude of hybrids of aerobics now on offer in health club studios.

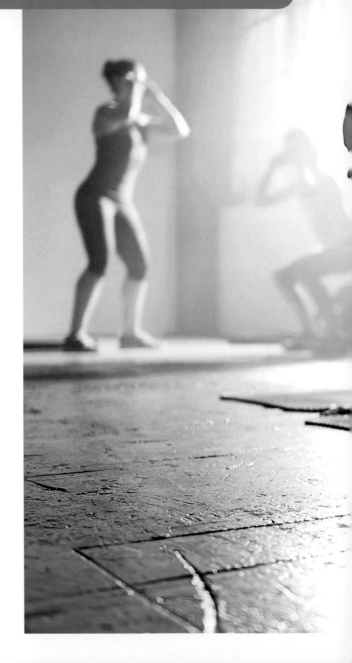

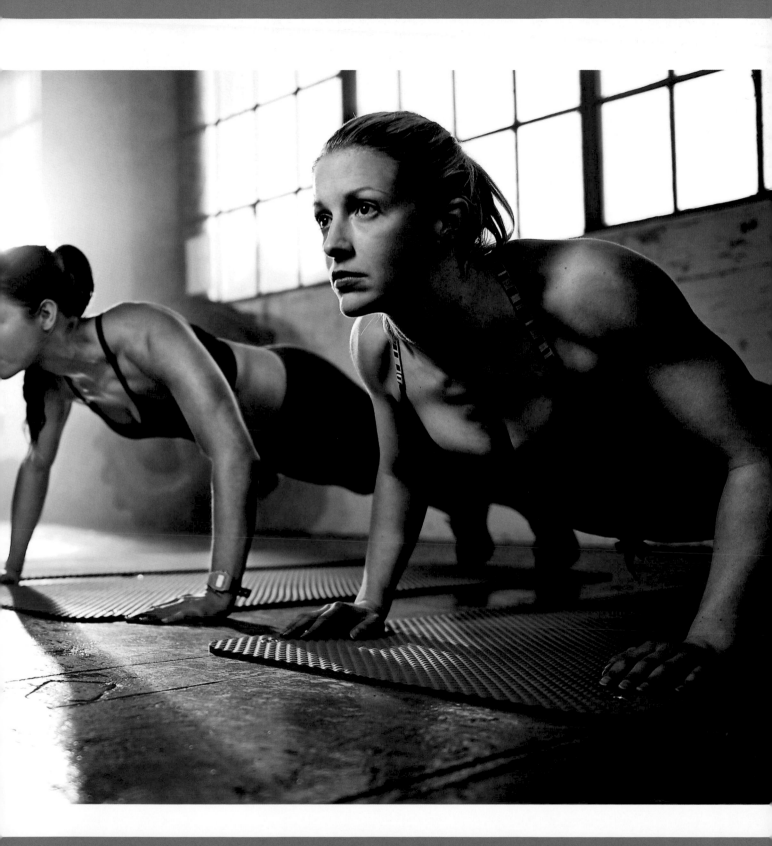

Women can also favour steady-state aerobic (cardiovascular, or 'CV') exercise, such as cycling, running and stepping, in an attempt to burn calories in the so-called 'fat-burning zone' (a concept that is challenged and in many ways incorrect). It often seems that the weights room, and in particular the free weights area with its dumbbells, barbells and kettlebells, is restricted to men, so not surprisingly you may feel intimidated should you want to enter this world.

I edited *ultra-FIT* magazine for over ten years and we had many features sent in and commissioned from and by women who were initially mistrusting of weights and what they perceived resistance training could do for them. They expressed thoughts such as, 'It'll bulk me up', 'I don't want to lose my curves', 'I don't want to become manly'..., yet by the end of their resistance journey they wondered why they had put it off for so long. They found that by using weights, they lost weight, shaped up, developed curves in the right places, improved their quality of life and zest and felt so much better. In this book you'll read testimonials from numerous women (of various backgrounds and with varying starting points) who have all succeeded with resistance training, in ways that exceeded their expectations.

As well as these testimonials, you'll also discover as you read some of the reasons – real, scientific ones – why resistance training is a must in your workouts. But don't worry, I'll cut through the jargon to provide you with the information you'll need as simply and practically as possible.

As a writer, editor, personal trainer and sports coach I have come into contact with some of the foremost training and nutrition experts and fitness brands in the world and have had the chance to pick brains and really understand whether what's being said is hot air or hot stuff! I certainly believe that the tips, strategies and plans provided in this book will get results. Our lives are continually time-poor and everything seems to come at us at a million miles an hour – consequently, you don't want to waste your workout time or follow some spurious weight-loss plan quickly lifted from social media or the web. Resistance training will boost your health and quality of life and have such a positive influence – but you need to do it properly.

This book takes you on a complete resistance training journey. The initial chapters inform on the numerous reasons to resistance train and the types and benefits of each. We'll then progress to how you can construct a relevant training programme, for example by considering training systems and training variables. In Chapters 4 and 5 you'll find a 24-week progressive workout programme (divided into different training blocks respectively). This programme introduces different exercise options and training systems, which are fully explained and illustrated by way of description and photographs.

In Chapter 7, we delve into the world of nutrition. Fuelling your body optimally is a must for good health and training adaptation, and – just as there are myths

> They found that by using weights, they lost weight, shaped up, developed curves in the right places, improved their quality of life and zest, and felt so much better.

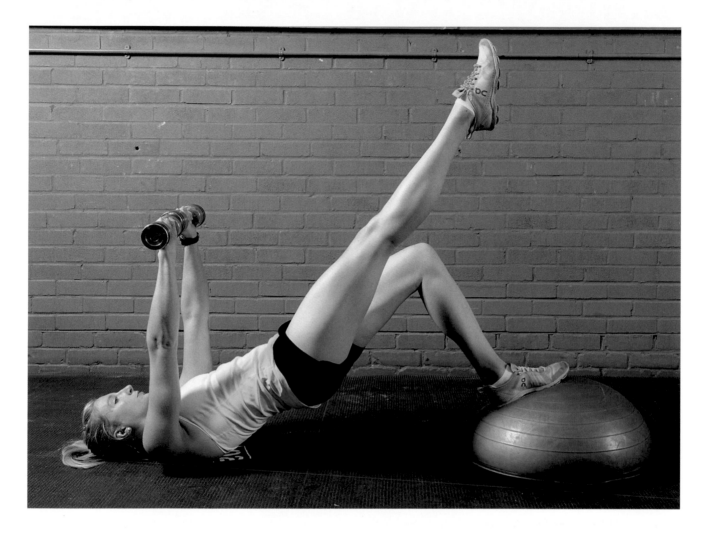

when it comes to resistance training – there are as many, if not more, when it comes to the 'best' diet. And, of course, without motivation you'll struggle to keep on the resistance training path. Chapter 8, therefore, provides some great ideas, thoughts and tips on how to stay positive and give yourself the best chance to work out and eat to achieve your best you.

I'd like to thank the numerous women (and men) who have contributed to this project over many years (you'll meet them as you turn from page to page). My editorial and fitness/sports training experience has enabled me to learn from, read, listen to and publish so many women's inspirational and life-changing stories.

By the end of *Strength Training for Women*, I hope you'll wonder why you ever resisted resistance training before.

John Shepherd

2 WHY WOMEN NEED RESISTANCE

Health benefits of resistance training

I'm now about to convince you why you need to resistance train! We'll first take a look at numerous health reasons and then move on to dispelling a few myths that seem to have entered workout folklore when it comes to women and weight training.

▶ Resistance training is 'feel good, look good' medicine

With ageng and increased inactivity comes a loss of muscle mass, which can range from 3 to 8 per cent per decade. You might not be alarmed by these figures, thinking that 'you don't want muscle anyway'. Well, with muscle loss comes a loss of strength, mobility and body shape, as well as poor posture. These negatives become more pronounced over time. So you might now want to rethink things. For inspiration, read what happened when Sonjia Ashby decided to get off the CV machines and lift heavier weights – see panel overleaf.

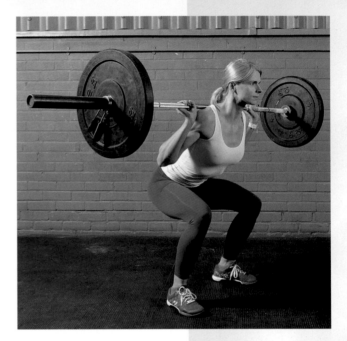

▲ Whether young or old, you will bolster your bones with weight training.

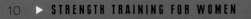

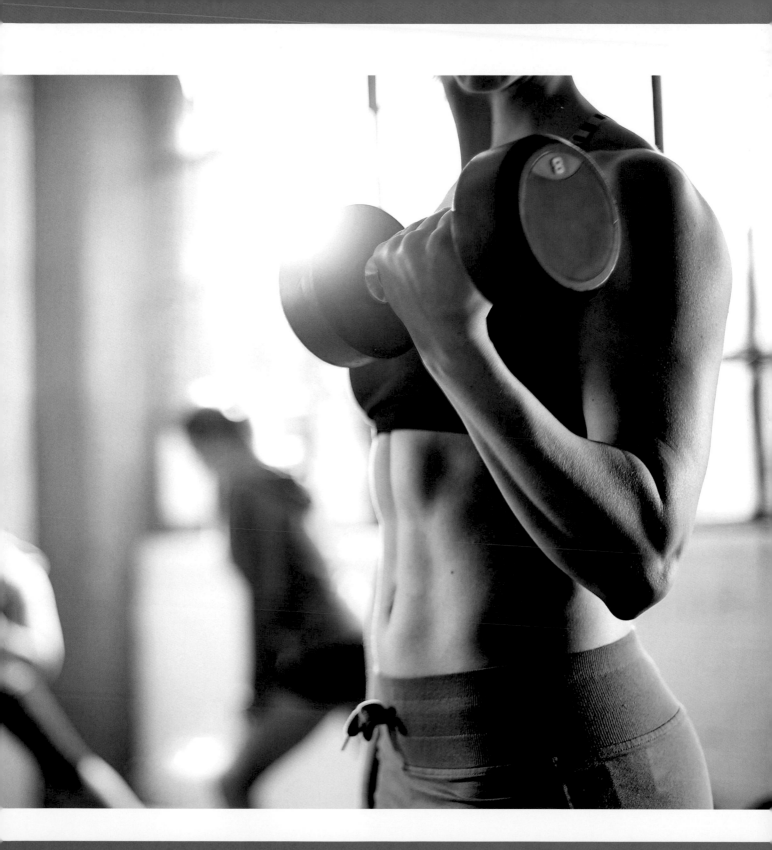

Sonjia Ashby

LIVING PROOF WHY YOU SHOULD RESISTANCE TRAIN

'It was in October 2012 when I changed my style of training. I had been doing Spinning® classes and other cardio sessions four or five times a week, together with a few weights. Then I changed to lifting heavy weights, training individual body parts and doing HIIT (High Intensity Interval Training) a few times a week. Why did I make the change? Well, I kept seeing other women on the Internet the same age as me and with children, living busy lives with amazing physiques. I researched what training they did to achieve their great bodies and discovered that lifting heavier (weights) was key to their lean shape and great proportions. So, that's why I changed my training to achieve my fitness goals.

'I'm now in the best shape of my life. I'm more confident, stronger and very happy. I totally enjoy the challenge of lifting heavy and the adrenalin buzz I get from it, and I have a personal trainer who helps me. I made this decision to ensure that I was lifting correctly. He also helped me to realise that there's a mindset behind lifting weights. The myth surrounding the belief that "if women lift weights, they will get bulky" really needs to be laid to rest because it's so not true! I'm proof and I'm just eight months into this training. So, I'd like to encourage women to step away from the cardio machines because they are taking you nowhere, and to lift proper weights instead!'

Follow Sonjia on her fitness journey on Facebook.

▶ Right: Sonjia Ashby

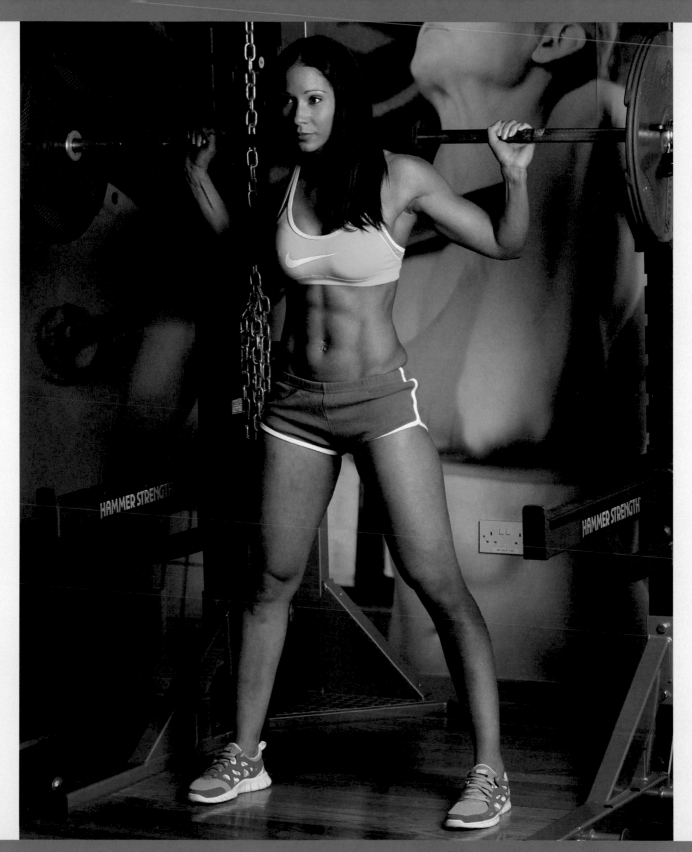

▶ Resistance training improves bone health – irrespective of age

With age, bones become thinner and weaken – this is something that has a more significant effect on women than men. Known as osteoporosis, this can make fractures all the more likely as decades pass. However, resistance training when young, throughout life and after menopause (of which more later) can make a big difference and significantly boost bone mass and slow down bone density decline. One study involving thirty 22-year-old women who completed 12 weeks of squat training using heavy weights (85-90 per cent of 1 rep max – that's the maximum you could lift only once) discovered that the women increased their hip bone mineral density by 1 per cent and their lumbar spine bone mineral density by 2.2 per cent.[1] Their 1 rep maximums incidentally increased by 97 per cent – so they got a lot stronger too!

POST-MENOPAUSE

A similar study with post-menopausal women produced equally positive results.[2] The women in this survey again squatted over a 12-week period and trained three times a week. The women improved their 1 rep max by a staggering 154 per cent and the bone density of their lower spine by 2.9 per cent and of their neck by 4.9 per cent. The sports scientists also discovered that markers of an increased potential for bone formation (serum P1NP/CTX) were boosted.

▶ Fat burning and resistance training

Cardiovascular (CV) exercise is not the only way to burn calories and fat. OK, chances are you will burn more calories going for a 30-minute run compared to a

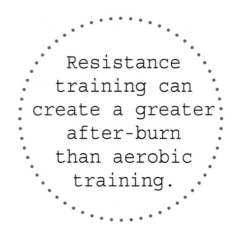

Resistance training can create a greater after-burn than aerobic training.

30-minute weights session; however, this fails to account for the effects of the workout on body composition – that's your fat to lean (muscle) ratio. There are also other crucial additional potential outcomes of resistance training, such as the hormonal response and enhanced post-workout calorie burning – of which more later. Muscle is metabolically active – the leaner you are, the more calories your body will burn. It's estimated that for every half a kg/1lb of lean muscle you gain, your body will burn 35–50 calories each and every day just to maintain it. Regular CV exercisers may lose weight but end up with a body that is less toned and can hold fat around key 'problem' areas, such as the abdomen and hips. Some research with older women backs this up: researchers discovered that weight training lowered body fat levels in women aged 60 plus. Over a 24-week period they increased their lean mass by 1.5kg (3½lb), which given their age was significant.[3]

As pointed out above, gaining lean weight as a consequence of resistance training can increase calorie burning and, more specifically, resting metabolic rate (RMR). RMR refers to the energy that is used while you are awake to maintain all essential bodily functions and accounts for 60–75 per cent of the calories you burn daily

– called Total Daily Energy Expenditure (see Chapter 7 for more detail). Here's some relevant research.[4] Fifteen women aged 50–69 participated in a 16-week survey. One group was of normal weight while the other group was overweight. Both groups resistance trained and both significantly increased their strength and their RMR. And for the overweight women, body fat, fat mass and percentage body fat were all equally significantly reduced. Proof that resistance training is a very effective weight loss training tool.

▶ Burning more calories with your feet up (sort of)!

When we exercise, our body uses more energy. Calories – mainly, although not exclusively, from carbohydrate – power our running, cycling and resistance training. In general, more calories will be burned when, for example, running for an hour as opposed to resistance training for an hour. However, the increased level of calorie burning does not just stop when we shower and head home from the gym. It's at this time, and beyond, that what is known as Excess Post-exercise Oxygen Consumption (EPOC) kicks in. More simply, this can be called the 'after-burn'. Research indicates that resistance training will create a greater after-burn than aerobic training. How so? There are two main periods of EPOC: one is created immediately after the workout and the other, although less intense, can last over a day. Although there can be great variation in terms of research results when calculating the extent of EPOC (due to factors such as the type and intensity of the workout and the age, gender and training experience of the subjects), there is still a significant amount of evidence that shows just how high metabolic rate can be elevated by resistance training. For example, one survey showed

UNDERSTANDING HORMONES, FAT BURNING AND SHAPING A GREAT BODY

Hormones are really like 'chemical messengers' in your body; they are produced by the endocrine system and endocrine glands, such as the hypothalamus in the brain. They run around in your body, busying themselves around your cells. The cell's actual response to a hormone is determined by the presence of certain protein receptors in its membrane or in its interior. Muscle fibres, like the rest of the body, are made from cells – thus the rate of hormonal production and the way the hormones interact with these (and the rest of the body's cellular structure) can significantly influence training adaptation and weight loss and fat burning. There is even research that indicates that young women weight trainers can produce more growth hormone (GH) than men. Don't be shocked – this is good for achieving a toned, strong and life-lasting body.

If GH and testosterone deliver the messages we want, cortisol doesn't. Rather like getting a big bill through the post, it causes stress. Cortisol levels can be elevated after aerobic and anaerobic CV workouts. Thus a workout programme that includes lots of CV workouts can up cortisol levels and work against developing the type of body that you may desire. Your muscles may actually shrink and be weakened by cortisol and its blunting effects on androgen production. CV workouts can also produce great quantities of free radicals – which can increase cellular damage.

that RMR in women was increased by 18.6 per cent two hours after a 45-minute resistance training workout compared to the non-exercising control group.

So, why does resistance training create a considerable EPOC and therefore have great fat-burning potential? When you resistance train, particularly with heavy weights (in excess of 75 per cent of 1RM) and with a short recovery between sets (less than a minute), you get a very intense workout and your body releases a significant level of hormones specific to boosting fat loss and lean muscle.[6]

Intensity is the key. Let's consider cardio. Research indicates that low-level CV training – scientifically set at less than 50 per cent of VO2max (that's the maximum amount of oxygen your body can use to supply energy) or moderate intensity (50–75 per cent VO2max) – will not significantly boost the after-burn. Paradoxically, these are the types of workouts commonly prescribed to women and often favoured when attempting to work out to lose body fat, the erroneously called 'fat-burning zone' workouts.

When you lift weights or do body weight exercises, two key hormones are released – growth hormone and testosterone (note: although the latter is the male sex hormone, it's also produced in women to a lesser extent). These hormones are androgens and they have a positive, stimulatory effect on the body. Not only are they great in terms of what derives from your workouts (leaning you up and giving you better shape and posture) but they can also give you more energy and even do wonders for your skin and hair and have a multitude of other consequences positive to health and vitality.

 ## You need to eat a lot to be lean

Many women (and men) who CV train predominantly underestimate how many calories they actually need to consume to maintain RMR and keep their bodies powered up. The same can also apply when you resistance train.

An average woman may need 2,000 calories a day to maintain her RMR. Now, just dealing with the extra activity created by regular exercise (resistance or otherwise), she may burn a further 600 calories a day (achievable for a 45-minute high-intensity resistance workout), which can increase EPOC immediately after the workout and – take note – for over a day afterwards or even longer (with regular and similar weekly workouts).

Calories will also be needed to fuel non-exercise activity and even to fuel up – at least 10 per cent of Total Daily Energy Expenditure (TDEE) is used when eating. So an active woman who is resistance (or aerobically/anaerobically CV) training regularly, may actually need closer to 3,000 calories a day, just to maintain her energy levels and maintain weight. Now, if this were combined with a calorie restricted diet, metabolic rate could be slowed and important metabolic processes compromised as the body will not get sufficient calories to maintain energy balance.

The body could lurch into starvation mode – even if you don't feel hungry. Starvation mode results in the body hanging on to every calorie it gets and not burning it, in fear that the next will be a long time coming. This is a genetic and historical legacy from our cavewoman days, when our prehistoric forebears had to go long periods without food. Another problem would be that of your body not getting enough of the vital micronutrients (vitamins and minerals) needed for health to optimally grow and regenerate due to compromised total food consumption, i.e. one that does not meet training-elevated metabolic needs.

So, it's very important not to underestimate your food needs when resistance (or other) training regularly and particularly at a high intensity. It's often the case that those who train optimally and eat a lot are also the leanest and most athletic and shapely. As I will discuss later, it may also be an idea to skew your diet in favour of a greater consumption of protein – rather than carbs – in order to assist with getting lean and shedding fat (see Chapter 7 for more info).

IN BRIEF: OTHER HEALTH BENEFITS OF RESISTANCE TRAINING

▶ Resistance training may assist prevention and management of Type 2 diabetes (this type of diabetes is often brought on by poor diet and a lack of exercise). It achieves this by, for example, decreasing body fat and improving insulin sensitivity.

▶ Resistance training can enhance CV health by lowering blood pressure and Low-Density Lipoprotein (so-called 'bad' cholesterol) and raising levels of High-Density Lipoprotein (so-called 'good' cholesterol).

▶ Resistance training may be effective for reducing low back pain and easing discomfort associated with arthritis.

▶ Like all exercise, resistance training produces 'feel-good' endorphins.

Myth Busting

▶ Resistance training myth busting

In the first part of this chapter, some pretty strong health and fitness reasons, coupled with scientific research, were provided as to why you should resistance train. Now some myths are dispelled. These are the types of myth you'll often encounter when it comes to resistance training – you may even *believe* some of them yourself.

▶ Myth 1: 'I'll bulk up if I do weight training.'

The reality is that women aren't genetically predisposed to gain large amounts of muscle. Women do, as noted, produce testosterone and its production can be increased as a result of working out. However, overall its effects are much smaller than those it has on men in terms of building muscle. This is primarily due to the reduced amount of muscle that women carry compared to men, as well as a more limited testosterone release. So building more muscle (irrespective of any hormonal training response) is always going to be much more limited compared to men. However, when lean muscle is created it can have very positive effects, as we will note later and throughout this book.

Myth 2: 'Cardio is only "good" for fat burning.'

Cardiovascular exercise is great for heart health and improving endurance and general fitness. However, it's unlikely to build muscle, as muscles (or more precisely specific muscle fibres) are not overloaded in the right way necessary to do this (see Chapter 3 for more detail). Rather it burns calories and these calories can come from fat, carbohydrate and our lean body tissue – the key constituent of which is protein. Our body is predominantly made up of fat and lean (muscle) tissue and water. Simply weighing yourself only records body mass i.e. how *heavy* you are. The scales are not able to distinguish between fat and lean tissue. Thus you could shape up with weights, for example, 'build' a better-looking body and end up weighing more than you did before you started weight training. This would be because you increased your lean weight and reduced your fat weight. A very positive outcome, but one that your scales alone would not indicate.

Getting rid of muscle and keeping fat just does not make sense, but if you only CV exercise that's what can happen. One of the obvious ways to understand this is to think of an Olympic marathon runner – they tend to be stick thin, with slight arms and legs. This is because of the amount of CV (specifically running) training they do and the way their body responds to it. The extensive training mileage will reduce muscle mass in areas that are not really required for marathon running, i.e. the arms, and will also potentially 'eat' into the protein content of muscles elsewhere for fuel. As mentioned previously, less muscle reduces metabolic rate. If a regular gym-goer only does cardiovascular workouts, for example, their fat-burning engine becomes a poor performer, increasing

the likelihood that excess calories will be stored as fat on the body as there is insufficient muscle to optimally burn those calories. A 1kg/2lb loss of muscle will result in an approximate 70 kcal drop in daily energy requirements. This means our aerobic-loving exerciser will lose muscle, potentially gain fat and may even look no better than they did before starting their exercise regime. The answer is to resistance train, build lean muscle and shape, and limit CV exercise to a sufficient amount for health benefits.

Myth 3: 'If I resistance train, I'll use very light weights and lots of reps to tone.'

Picking up the smallest dumbbells and doing endless reps is not going to burn fat and shape figure-enhancing muscles.

To increase the size of a muscle, you need to target the 'right' muscle fibres – these are fast twitch muscle fibres. Don't worry, you're not going to fidget all day after doing a workout that specifically targets these (workouts that require a heavy weight to be tackled, for example). Rather you will increase the power, strength and size of these fibres due to the resistance you overcome and it's these changes that will create a better fat-burning body with a better lean muscle to fat ratio.

Performing lots and lots of dumbbell curls will have very little effect on actually toning your body, because this type of workout 1) targets the muscle fibres (specifically slow twitch fibres) that do not produce greater calorie-burning muscles and 2) does not in itself burn a substantial number of calories. It's a low energy workout and the outcome is equally low when it comes to building a lean, toned body, optimised for fat burning 24/7, long-term. However, much more intense workouts with body weight and lighter/medium weights with short recoveries (circuit training and

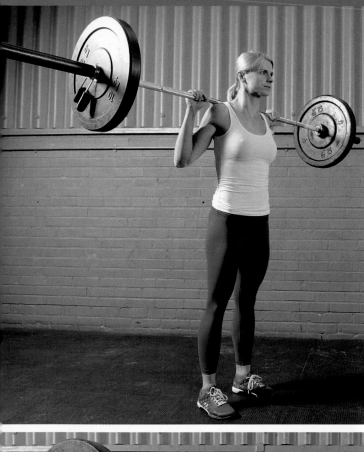

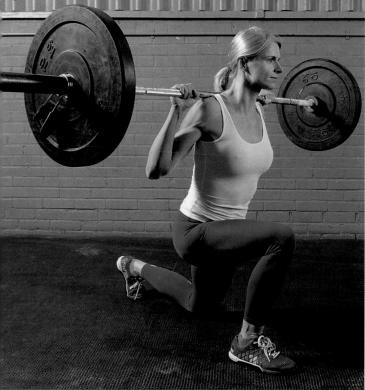

circuit resistance training, for example) can be much more beneficial. Such workouts will also produce a substantial EPOC and therefore after-burning of calories.

▶ Myth 4: 'If I do lots of triceps curls I'll banish my bingo wings.'

This myth follows on from the previous one. There's very little scientific evidence to suggest that exercising one body part with lots and lots of reps will reduce the fat around that body part (known as 'spot reduction'). What actually counts is total calorie burn and the use of exercises (and specific training systems – see Chapter 3) that have the greatest metabolic cost, i.e. they burn the most calories. Exercises that work a lot of muscles across a number of the body's joints offer the big pay-off. These are known as compound exercises and include the likes of squats and lunges and jumping exercises. Ten lunges performed with a heavy weight over three sets is going to have a far greater metabolic cost (short-term and long-term EPOC), calorie burning and positive body shaping outcome than 4 x 20 very light weight triceps curls. The same principle applies to ab exercises, where it's the resistance you overcome (the amount of 'overload') and not the number of reps you complete that will strengthen your core. Thus good technique, really focusing on the abdominals and 'squeezing' out reps, is far more advantageous than banging out hundreds of reps that use momentum supplied by the arms, for example, to create the movement.

◀ Go heavier – 3 x 10 lunges with a heavy weight will have a far greater after-burn than 4 x 20 triceps curls with a very light weight.

The body can't specify where fat (i.e. excess body weight) will be burned. When calories are burned and a positive energy balance is created (i.e. you burn more calories than you consume) then weight will be lost in general. Having said that, fat tends to be reduced first in areas of its greatest concentration, i.e. hips, thighs and abdomen. Stubborn areas of accumulation left after a training and nutrition programme, for example around the lower tummy, will often be difficult to lose and it's at those times that you need to alter your training to continually shock your system and create different training/fat-burning conditions – lots of relevant options are contained in Chapters 4, 5 and 6, the practical workout chapters of this book.

▶ Myth 5: 'Free weights are not free for women (because they're for men!).'

Perhaps this is not such a myth as it was a decade or so ago. Lifting barbells and kettlebells and using a Smith machine (a structure that supports and controls the path of a barbell), for example, have been seen as 'male only' activities, while women used fixed weight machines (and lighter free weights) or did dance classes instead of venturing into the free weights area of the gym. Again, the myth is based on the belief that free weights and heavier weights will build a manly physique and as I've indicated previously this is just not the case. Stereotyping is at play here and both genders would often consciously and unconsciously live up to these.

Delving into this myth a little further – many gyms have inner and outer thigh machines (for the adductor and abductor muscles respectively). These were the machines that you could virtually guarantee would not be used by men. Women, however, would do so in large numbers,

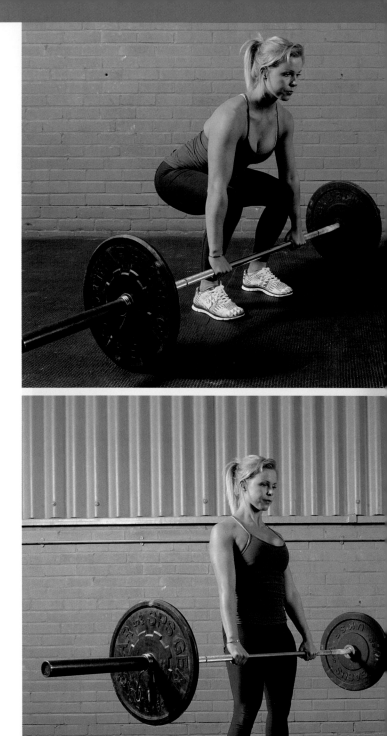

in the belief that they would banish cellulite and shape slender legs; the reality is far from this, as medium to heavy load squats or lunges or dead lifts (see Chapters 4 and 5) have far greater potential to shape the legs and bottom in the way most women want. It's the metabolic cost and compound nature of the free weight exercises mentioned that counts, and the way they build lean and shapely muscle curves.

Myth 6: 'When you stop training your muscle turns to fat.'

Muscle and fat are biologically different and cannot turn into each other. I've mentioned that muscle is metabolically active and a calorie burner, so if you stop training and don't also reduce what you eat (your calories 'in'), your muscle mass will decline as it is not being stimulated by relevant training, and you'll gain weight due to consuming too many calories.

Myth 7: 'I'll start to look masculine if I lift weights.'

The counter to this myth is very similar to that of the first, 1in that your body is not designed like a man's to build large muscles easily. The reality is that a carefully planned resistance and weight training programme can shape a great looking, toned and functional physique. Read the numerous testimonies that appear in this book and take a look at the accompanying images to see living proof that you should *not* offer resistance when it comes to resistance training!

◄ If you want great legs and bottom, then squat and dead lift.

3 THE PATH TO A GREAT BODY REQUIRES RESISTANCE

Understanding why and training systems

If I have done my job well so far, you should by now know the many positive benefits resistance training has for you, your body and your health. I'll also have dispelled some myths that may have been holding you back. In this chapter, we go into detail about resistance training and explain the different types and what they can do for health, fitness, fat burning and body shaping. We'll also identify the different training systems used in this book, which you can use yourself to construct different workouts in future, and training variables, which can affect the outcome of your workouts in so many ways. There'll be more on how your body adapts to resistance training and we'll also take a look at body type and body shape and how best to train accordingly against these.

▶ Body image

In our image-obsessed age, we are all concerned about how we look. Many of us, regardless of our gender, are dissatisfied with what we see in the mirror. Yes, men are increasingly feeling the same, but we may shrug off concerns about our body image or even overestimate our attractiveness – now, there's a thing! However, as a woman you'll probably feel that you are judged much

▶ There are so many different ways to resistence train - this chapter explains the benefits of many of them.

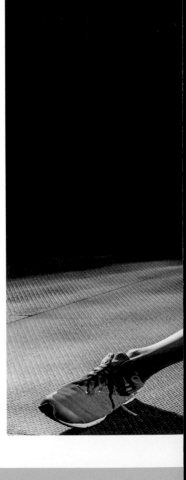

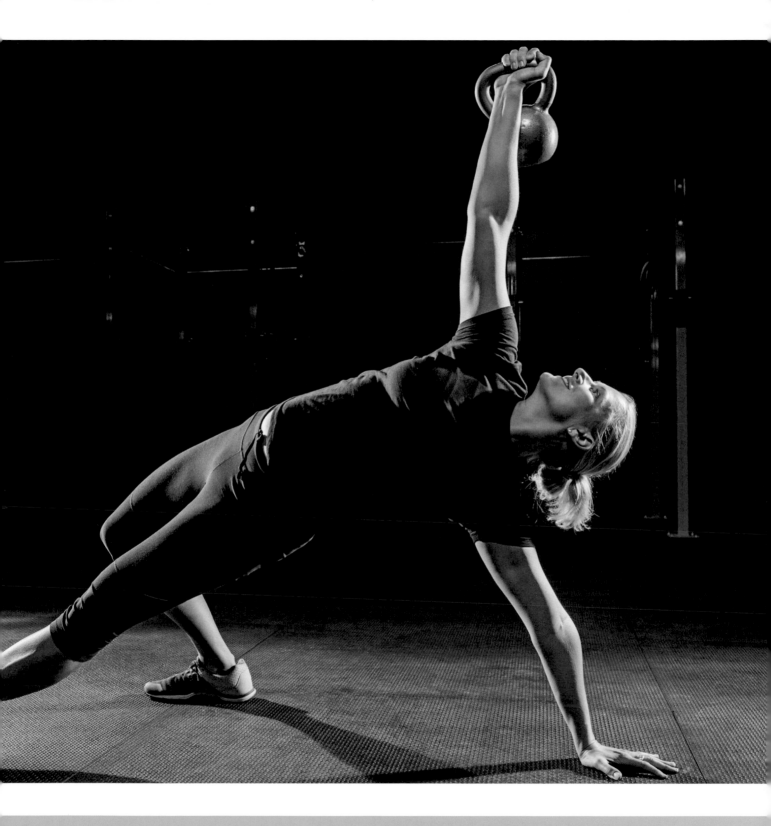

more on appearance. Consistent dissatisfaction with how you look is known as body dysmorphia and surveys show that girls as young as ten and under have dieted and can suffer from this. So when it comes to resistance training it's crucial that you see it as a means to improve your strength, health, well-being, fitness, functional movement and appearance. Embrace working out for these reasons and don't just lift weights, for example, to attempt to fulfil a somewhat skewed view of what the ideal woman (and not the ideal you) should look like. *Your* resistance-trained body *will* make *you* feel, look and move so much better. And – as the case studies show in this book – it will give you a lot more confidence, too.

▶ The difference between body type and body shape

There are three main body types, specifically known as somatotypes. These are: ectomorph, mesomorph and endomorph. The types can be described in more basic terms as: slim, athletic and rounder. This basic classification derives from the work of the psychologist William Sheldon and his work in the mid 20th century. Sheldon believed that each type had distinct physiological (and psychological) traits. Although his work is perhaps overstated, it does provide a valuable starting point for body type analysis. This is because it's possible to identify the ways in which each type typically responds to training and diet – thus potentially maximising training and dietary returns.

Most people are actually an amalgamation of the three body types and there is a further level of somatotype classification that describes a body type in terms of parts of the three. This is known as 'dominant somatotype'. Sheldon in fact identified seven parts (1–7) for each

somatotype, with 1 being the minimum and 7 the maximum number of parts attributable to that somatotype. For example, '2–6–3' indicates 'low endomorphy-high mesomorphy-low ectomorphy'. This would be a body type that resembled, for example, someone like Jessica Ennis-Hill.

Your body shape results from how you work out, your diet and your lifestyle, while your body type is a determinant of your genetics. A long distance runner, for example, may have a body type that has mesomorphic tendencies; however, while they are in training, due to their high calorific needs and a lack of training emphasis on building (and maintaining muscle), they develop a more ectomorphic shape. As indicated, this can also happen to the bodies of the many women who believe that CV training is the only way to burn fat and shape up. On the flip side, countless millions will take on much more of an endomorphic shape as they gain weight due to a lack of exercise and excessive and poor food choices – as illustrated by the current levels of obesity in the western world.

BODY SHAPE

In Table 1 you'll find some information on typical body shapes. Body shape is probably a more realistic starting point than body type, as it's the one that is influenced the most through diet, exercise and lifestyle – although it is important to note that your body type lies beneath this. Somewhat obviously and relevantly, it's also literally 'the shape you are in'.

Consider the information presented for the four shapes, as knowing how your body is likely to respond to training (resistance or otherwise) will help you to optimise your workouts and better understand how to get the most from your training. Having said that, it's important to note that no two bodies are the same or will respond in an identical way

Body Shapes

TABLE 1

APPLE	PEAR	HOURGLASS	CELERY
Tends to carry weight around abdomen	Weight stored around hips, bottom and thighs	Shoulders and hips are similar width	Shoulders, waist and hips are of similar width
Bottom is small but flat	Often has slim waist and flat stomach	Curvy figure with full chest, but in proportion	Tends to have a 'straight up and down' appearance
Can have delicate wrists and ankles	Typically narrow shoulders	Tends to lose and gain weight evenly	Can have a boyish look, due to lack of curves
Best feature – slim hips and good legs	**Best feature** – nicely defined back and slim arms	**Best feature** – shapely waist	**Best feature** – long lean legs
Generous chest but can be out of proportion	Tends to lose weight from face and upper body	Bottom and hips may appear wide	Tends to lose weight evenly
Larger chest and stomach can make for a rounded look	Often appears to have rounded shoulders	Upper arms may become fleshy	Chest tends to be relatively flat

to training and/or diet. Over time, you should be able to understand what works for your shape and type.

▶ Train your shape – advanced considerations

Although it is the aim of this book to provide a full vindication for the inclusion of resistance training, it is important to consider certain thoughts on body shaping, particularly for those who specifically want to change/balance their body type/shape. As you will see from the information on somatotype and body shape, your training response can be influenced by what type you are. You also need to appreciate the intricacies of fat burning and how fat can't be trained away from one body site by selected exercises ('spot reduction'). And you need to throw into all of this the benefits of increased lean muscle for fat burning on an everyday basis due to an increased metabolic rate. The workouts that follow in Chapters 4 and 5 are designed to develop the optimum lean, fat-burning body, one that is strong and functional. It is beyond the scope of this book to go into great detail about targeting specific muscle groups with relevant exercises and loadings (the weight on the bar/machine and so on) to shape and balance the proportions of your body shape. What do I mean by this? Here's an example. If you are a pear shape, then working your upper back and front and rear shoulders, with exercises such as shoulder presses and various rowing movements, can add extra size to the muscles there and thus help to balance your body. You might also want to reduce the amount of lower body work you do to minimise size gain there. Once you understand how to train, you'll be able to adapt and design training programmes that are more related to your specific shape, should you wish.

YOU CANNOT SPOT REDUCE

I want to make it very clear that training one muscle or muscle group only is not solely going to have an effect on that muscle. Any increase in lean muscle by way of resistance training will increase metabolic rate, whether it be in the arms or the legs. Thus, targeting your bottom with squats, for example, to add shape will up your body's overall calorie burning through potential gains in lean muscles and fat could be lost as a result from any other body part. Now, that's no bad thing! Do, however, remember that your body shape may have an influence on the response you get to your training.

BODY SHAPE CONSIDERATIONS

A celery shape, for example, will tend to have more difficulty building lean muscle due to her physiology and should really focus on compound movements for the lower body with exercises such as squats and lunges, with heavy weights (once sufficient condition has been established), and keep any CV work to a real minimum.

An hourglass shape will usually respond quite quickly to all types of training. It may therefore be necessary to change training regimes more regularly to ensure continued training improvements. It's also important to see where changes are occurring in body shape and to keep these balanced across the whole body. This could mean for example reducing the amount of leg work done for a while.

Apple shapes can benefit from HIT training to create an increased metabolic rate that can help shift abdominal fat. They may also create more symmetry by working on their shoulder muscles to create greater balance for the top of their frame. Similarly consistent use of compound lower body exercises may also help to create greater balance.

A pear shape with rounded shoulders, as indicated,

would benefit from upper back and rear shoulder exercises, such as various types of rowing exercises, to improve the strength of these muscles. Doing this will 'pull' the shoulders back and improve posture.

⊞ Not all strength is the same!

▶ Strength types

The way you overcome resistance in your workouts will specifically affect the type of strength you develop and the way your muscles respond, together with the way your body shapes up.

As well as the weight on barbells and dumbbells, there are many other variables in terms of the way you overcome resistance – for example, resistance can be increased by using a steeper body angle, or shorter or longer strap for many suspension trainer exercises, or by employing different training systems, varying the number of repetitions, recoveries and sets you use and even the speed at which you perform an exercise (the lifting and lowering parts).

Table 2 provides an overview of strength types. You'll see from the training programmes later on in this book that they overlap and develop these different types as you progress your resistance training. In Chapter 4, for example, the first four weeks of the 24-week programme build a background of relevant strength and emphasise what's known as 'strength endurance', while the later weeks (5–12) focus more on using greater resistance and increasing lean muscle mass, resulting in greater potential for specific fat burning.

In Chapter 5, where you'll find a further 12-week training plan, different exercises and further training systems are introduced to continue the process of developing a great, fit, functional and toned resistance-trained body. The main change in this part of the plan is the move to heavier weights.

The programmes in this book follow a periodised approach to training – this means that each week, collection of weeks and months of training build progressively on the workouts performed in the previous one/ones. Doing this creates the best conditions for your body to adapt systematically, progressively and safely. Sometimes training can be haphazard and this unsurprisingly gets haphazard results – so we want to avoid that. It's also an aim of this book to enable you to acquire the skills necessary to develop your own training plans, perhaps so you can adjust the workouts to account for your particular body shape/body type or even so that you can plan your own workouts fully in future after completing the programme in the book. If you understand what an exercise and a workout and training plan is designed to do, then it's all the more likely that it will be successful and I very much hope that you will develop that level of understanding as you read and progress through the chapters.

> If you understand what an exercise and a workout and training plan is designed to do then it's all the more likely that it will be successful

Different strength types and how to train for them

TABLE 2

STRENGTH TYPE	PRIMARY PURPOSE AND MUSCLE FIBRES TARGETED	MOST COMMONLY USED WEIGHT TRAINING SYSTEM	RESISTANCE TRAINING AND FITNESS, EVERYDAY AND SPORTS BENEFITS
Strength endurance	• To develop muscles' ability to produce repeated contractions under conditions of fatigue. Targets 'slow twitch' muscle fibre (and 'transitional fast twitch' fibres). • To create a base on which to build workouts that are more demanding, strength-wise. • Strength endurance training is unlikely to increase muscle size but can create a sizeable after-burn.	• High reps, for example 15 plus, with light added resistances – 30–50% 1RM* • Simple sets • Supersets • EDT • CT • CRT • Drop sets • AMRAP	• Great for creating a foundation on which to build greater power and maximum strength, which will develop your body's ability to become a better fat-burning machine. • Field sports, rowing, martial arts, climbing, cycling, triathlon, hiking. • Like all resistance training, this will benefit everyday activities, such as lifting objects, walking and climbing stairs.
Power (a measure of 'strength x speed' – the more you have, the faster you will run, for example)	• To enable fast and powerful movements to be produced. Targets 'fast twitch' muscle fibre.	• Medium reps, for example 6–10, with medium to heavy loadings – 70–80% 1RM* • Simple sets • Supersets • Pyramids • Split routines	• Great for boosting the muscle-building hormones, which can stimulate lean muscle growth. • Virtually all sports will benefit from such power training – for example, running and sprinting, netball, football and hockey.
Maximum strength	• To develop the strength required to exert high levels of muscular force. This strength type will almost exclusively target 'fast twitch' muscle fibres.	• Low reps, for example 1–5, with heavy loading – 80–100% 1RM* • Simple sets • Pyramids • Split routines • Negatives	• As noted, this will develop your ability to overcome heavy resistances. It can build shape and strength. • Maximum strength is needed by all athletes, from runners and triathletes to field sports players and sprinters, for example.
Increased muscle mass ('size with strength')	• To increase muscle size and develop 'fast twitch' muscle fibre.	• Medium to high reps, for example 8–12, with medium to heavy loading – 70–80% plus of 1RM* • Simple sets • Supersets • Pre-exhaust • Drop sets	• 'Size with strength' is a very intense method of training that considerably stimulates the muscle building hormones. This type of training is ideal for those seeking quick gains in lean muscle.

Some of the terminology used in Table 2 is subsequently explained in Table 4 (Training Systems).
* 1RM means one repetition maximum – the maximum amount of weight you could lift in one lift. As a simple example, if your maximum squat is 100kg (220lb) then 70 per cent would be 70kg (154lb). Knowing your 1RM is important in terms of ensuring that the specific outcomes of a resistance training workout are achieved. Ways to calculate your rep maximums are provided later (see Calculating your 1 Repetition Maximum, below).

CALCULATING YOUR 1 REPETITION MAXIMUM (1RM)

There are various ways to calculate your 1RM; you need to do this so you can maximise the returns from strength, fitness, sports training (if desired) and body shape. The most basic method is to load as much weight as you can on to a bar or machine and simply see if you can move it. Note that this should be attempted by experienced weight trainers only, with extreme caution. The information in the following chart will give you an idea of the estimated percentage of 1RM in terms of the number of reps you can perform on weight training exercises. Note that these repetition maximums can vary according to the exercise being performed, your training experience, the stage in your training and your willpower.

CALCULATE YOUR 1RM
You can also use this formula to calculate your 1RM:
Reps x weight x 0.0333 + weight
So if you manage 6 reps at 70kg (154lb):
6 x 70 = 420 x 0.0333 = 13.98 + 70; estimated 1RM = 83.98kg (185lb)
There are also a number of apps available that calculate your 1RM in a similar way, for example 1 Rep Max Calculator.

NOTE: your 1RM will not remain the same and therefore to get the maximum from your workouts you should retest/recalculate from time to time. I would suggest every 4–6 weeks. Make sure you are rested before performing such a physical test and that you are familiar with the exercises you are going to perform. Have a training partner on hand to assist should you need help completing an exercise.

%1RM	Maximum Repetitions
100	1
95	2
93	3
90	4
87	5
85	6
83	7
80	8
77	9
75	10
70	11
67	12
60	15

Knowing your muscles

Your body has, on average, 36 per cent muscle (men average 42 per cent). The key ingredient of muscle is protein.

There are more than 430 muscles in the body that we can control. These are known as voluntary muscles. To move a voluntary muscle, the brain sends an electrical signal to the muscle/muscles. This turns the key to 'switch on' the muscle/muscles. Carbohydrate in particular, as well as fat, specific body chemicals and oxygen, supply the fuel to make muscles move. Muscles can only pull on bones, but they do this by way of different muscular actions, of which more later.

Muscles are composed of different fibre types and these reflect the function they are designed for, i.e. to produce continuous (endurance) type movements or stronger, more powerful and faster, short-lived ones. As indicated, these are known as 'slow twitch' and 'fast twitch' fibres and are stimulated by different types of resistance training methods and loads (i.e. weight on a barbell). This affects the specific 'strength type' developed. For example, if you consistently train for power and maximum strength, targeting your fast twitch muscle fibres, you will become stronger, more powerful and quicker and at the same time develop a body that's metabolically active (i.e. good at burning calories) – this is a result of increased muscle.

The Major Muscle Groups   TABLE 3

MAJOR MUSCLE GROUP	INDIVIDUAL MUSCLES
Calves	Gastrocnemius and soleus
Thighs	Quadriceps (front) and hamstrings (back) Adductors (inside) Abductors (outside)
Bottom	Gluteus maximus (behind) Gluteus medius (sides of hips)
Pelvic area	Hip flexors (muscles at top of thighs)
Back	Latissimus dorsi (sides of back), rhomboids (central upper back), trapezius (sides of neck into upper back), erector spinae (lower back muscles)
Abdomen	Rectus abdominis (main front muscle), obliques (side muscles)
Chest	Pectorals
Shoulders	Deltoids
Upper arms	Biceps (front) and triceps (back)

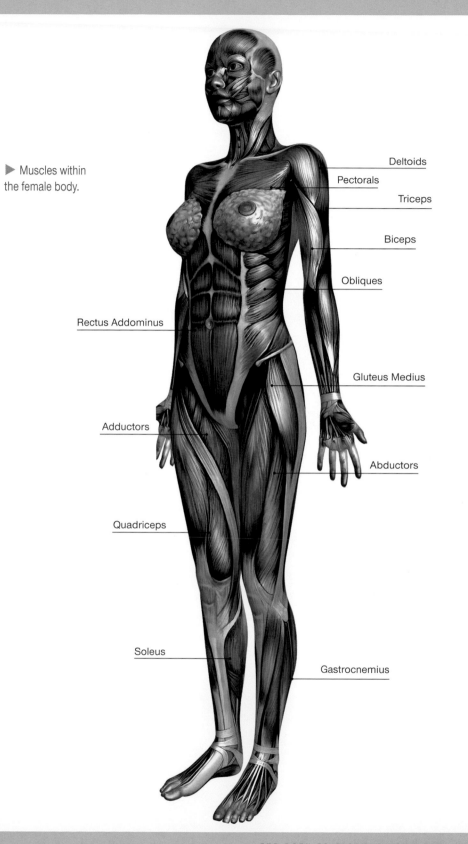

▶ Muscles within the female body.

Deltoids

Pectorals

Triceps

Biceps

Obliques

Rectus Addominus

Gluteus Medius

Adductors

Abductors

Quadriceps

Soleus

Gastrocnemius

Are women's muscles different to men's?

No, 'muscle is muscle'. Men have more, as explained, and it's this that gives them greater overall strength.

A research study found that women had 52 per cent and 66 per cent of the strength of men in the upper arms (biceps) and thighs (quadriceps) respectively. However, when the size of the muscles was taken into account, the level of strength between men and women was more or less the same. A bigger muscle is able to produce more force than a smaller one.

However, the researchers discovered that men's muscle fibres are larger than women's – this shows that it's likely for men to bulk up through resistance training, but not women.[8]

▼ Women's muscles are the same as men's.

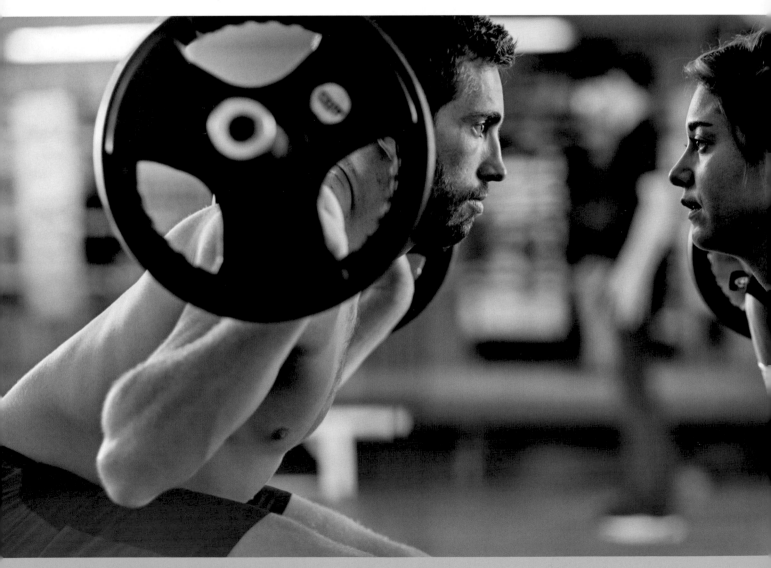

▶ Muscle fibre – in brief
'FAST TWITCH' MUSCLE FIBRE

Fast twitch muscle fibre:

▶ develops in response to medium to heavy levels of resistance.

▶ develops in response to sprinting and jumping exercises.

▶ requires you to be in the 'zone' (mentally focused) to maximise its response because you need to supply

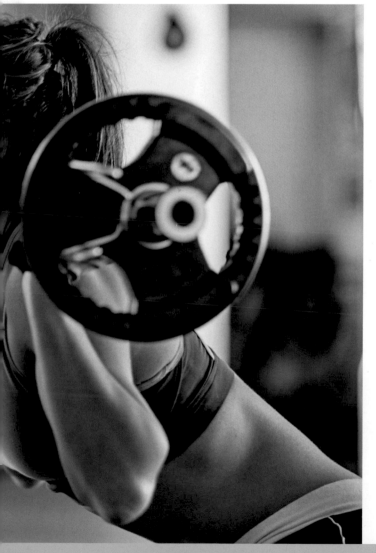

sufficient neural energy to power up these fibres. If you don't have that focus, they won't respond.

▶ relies on the anaerobic energy system for power.

▶ increases the body's calorie burning potential as a result of creating additional lean muscle mass.

There are two types of fast twitch muscle fibre – 2a and 2b. The former is also known as 'intermediate', as the fibres can develop either greater endurance or speed, strength and power with the appropriate training. However, type 2b fibres are designed for optimum speed and strength and can only be targeted by medium to heavy levels of resistance, i.e. weights in excess of 85 per cent 1 rep max, and power exercises such as sprinting and jumping.

'SLOW TWITCH' MUSCLE FIBRE

Slow twitch muscle fibre:

▶ develops in response to light to medium levels of resistance – muscular endurance results.

▶ develops in response to continuous endurance type activities such as running, cycling and swimming.

▶ requires less mental energy to sustain moderate intensity efforts.

▶ relies on the aerobic energy system for power.

▶ is unlikely to increase in size and therefore improve the body's fat burning potential.

An overemphasis on CV activities, which target slow twitch muscle fibre, can reduce the calorie burning effectiveness of the body by reducing muscle mass and thus calorie burning potential.

Muscular actions

Our muscles can generate force in different ways.

ISOTONIC MUSCULAR ACTION ▶

When you walk, run, jump, turn or make any of thousands of other possible movements, muscles work isotonically – this involves a concentric and eccentric action.

ECCENTRIC MUSCULAR ACTION

An eccentric muscular action occurs when a muscle lengthens under load. During a dumbbell curl, the biceps muscle extends eccentrically under load to lower the weight. The same happens to the muscles at the front of your thighs (the quadriceps) when you walk or step into a lunge.

▼

◀ CONCENTRIC MUSCULAR ACTION

A concentric muscular action happens when a muscle shortens under load. It's the most common of all muscular actions (fitness and everyday). A typical example is when you curl a kettlebell – in doing so, the biceps muscle works concentrically.

ISOMETRIC MUSCULAR ACTION ▶

During an isometric movement, no movement actually occurs – you hold your limbs or your body in place by the action of muscles working against each other (or against a machine/immovable object). Isometric muscular action is crucial in exercises such as the core-developing plank and is also involved in everyday activities, such as sitting and standing.

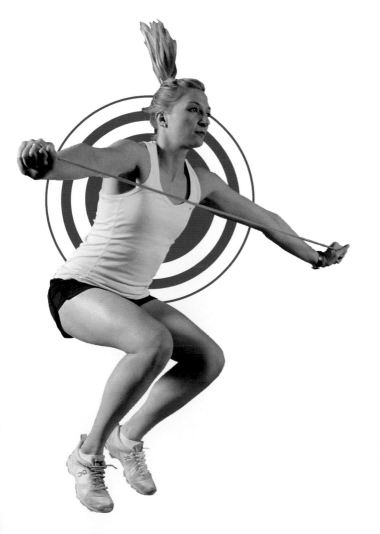

◀ PLYOMETRIC MUSCULAR ACTION

A plyometric movement involves the stretching of a muscle/muscles and then an immediate, rapid shortening (specifically, an eccentric muscular action followed by a concentric one). This produces more power than would be possible either eccentrically or concentrically because the stretch primes the subsequent muscle shortening action. It's a bit like pulling out a spring to its maximum length (the eccentric muscular action) and then letting it go – the spring will snap back (the concentric muscular action) very quickly, releasing a high level of energy/power. Plyometrics are therefore also called 'stretch/reflex' or 'elastic' strength exercises.

Plyometric exercises are great to include in your training programme and are often found in High Intensity Training (HIT) workouts and the world of the recent fitness phenomenon CrossFit®. You'll find examples in Chapters 4, 5 and 6. They have a high metabolic cost and are therefore very beneficial in terms of calorie burning and targeting fast twitch muscle fibre, thus creating the right conditions for increasing your body's lean muscle mass.

GETTING THE BENEFITS OF YOUR TRAINING

▶ Whatever the training method, i.e. resistance or CV based, it's in the time when you are *not* training that your muscles (including your heart) develop increased strength, strength endurance and power. Specifically in resistance training, muscle protein is broken down as a result of the training and it's in the downtime between your workouts that muscles rebuild and grow stronger/increase in size.

▶ Adaptation is crucial to fitness and condition improvements – if you always do what you've always done, you'll get the same results. Consequentially, you need to cycle your training and use different exercises and training systems to optimise your progression. The workout programmes in Chapters 4 and 5 do just this. And because of this it's important to realise that more training will not necessarily result in more strength and lean muscle mass gains. Too much training can actually be counterproductive and reduce the potential positive results as your mind, muscles and body become overtrained and less responsive.

▶ DOMS is the pain and stiffness felt in muscles several hours after exercise.

Muscle soreness

Pushing through barriers, using a new resistance training system or returning to exercise after a layoff can leave your muscles sore. This can vary from a little discomfort and stiffness to muscles that feel heavy and tender to the touch. This soreness is known as 'Delayed Onset of Muscle Soreness' (DOMS). The mechanisms behind DOMS are not fully understood but it appears that the stimulus (workout/exercise) produces microscopic tears in the muscles, causing the soreness. These need recovery time and optimum nutrition (see Chapter 7) to heal and for the soreness to go. It's the recovery that results in positive muscular adaptation.

Some soreness is actually an indication of a positive muscular response – it indicates that you have pushed your muscles beyond previous limits and that they have adapted, or rather will adapt, positively in response.

Eccentric muscular actions seem to create greater muscle soreness than concentric ones. However, once recovered your muscles will be unlikely to suffer from a similar bout of soreness, as long as you maintain similar training.

Energy systems

Our bodies produce energy in two basic ways – aerobically (with oxygen) or anaerobically (without oxygen, of which there are two systems). Resistance training is primarily an anaerobic activity, as you'll only be lifting weights or working against the resistance of a suspension trainer for a relatively short period of time, usually a matter of seconds. The energy required to power these movements comes from stored chemicals, such as creatine phosphate. There are exceptions – for example, if you were completing a circuit training session (with body weight and/or weights exercises) on a relatively continuous basis for, say, 20 minutes; the session could comprise 30-second work periods and 30-second rest periods. Thus your heart rate would be elevated and would remain so throughout the workout, which would mean that you would be working aerobically to sustain your energy levels. The emphasis of the 24-weeks' worth of workouts in this book (see Chapters 4 and 5) resides firmly on the anaerobic side of the energy equation.

ENERGY SYSTEMS — TABLE 4

System	Duration	Oxygen reliance	Typical training activity
Aerobic	90sec and above	Total	Continuous, low to moderate intensity activity, i.e. running and cycling
Short-term anaerobic	8–10sec–90sec	Minor initially but increases rapidly	Fast and continuous effort – for example, a 500m sprint
Immediate anaerobic	8–10sec	None	Resistance training – for example, low-volume reps of exercises (3–12) performed with 30sec-plus recoveries between, 40m sprints. Most plyometric exercises

Mental energy

As I mentioned when talking about strength types, the power and maximum-strength exercises in particular require you to 'commit' in order to get the best out of them. What do I mean? Well, when attempting to lift a weight at or around 80 per cent of your 1 rep max, unless you want to lift the weight, you won't. It's a bit like twisting a stubborn lid off a bottle – you draw breath and really focus your energy on moving the lid and you will twist it off. Focus gets the mental energy needed from your brain to your muscles to loosen the cap and it's the same when it comes to resistance training – focus, and you'll overcome resistance.

MENTAL FATIGUE

Rather like physical energy, you don't have an infinite amount of mental energy. Perhaps you have noticed that, when you do a resistance training workout, you perform the first few exercises much better than the ones you finish with – this is particularly so if you are using heavy weights. Your mental energy begins to wane and you may not be able to attack exercises and sets as your workout progresses. It's important to be aware of this because 1) if you continue to train session after session at a high intensity with insufficient recoveries you run the risk of overtraining, and 2) your injury risk can be increased if you perform exercises with fatigue. Quality is much more important than quantity in resistance training, especially when trying to develop a lean body; it's far better to reduce the number of sets or reps you perform and keep up the required intensity, rather than push through and run the risk of training at an intensity that will not get the results being targeted. This is especially the case with the latter phases of the programme, particularly the last 12 weeks in Chapter 5. This is when the sessions become much more intense. With these workouts, you simply won't be able to move the weights required if you lack the mental energy to do so.

BRACE YOUR CORE

Incidentally, drawing breath and firming up your core, as you would when attempting to loosen a stubborn lid, allows you to generate more power. You can do something similar when weight training, using a technique known as creating 'Intra-abdominal Pressure' (IAP, see page 47). IAP can boost strength and power outputs and also make your core much more resilient and less likely to be injured when performing certain resistance exercises.

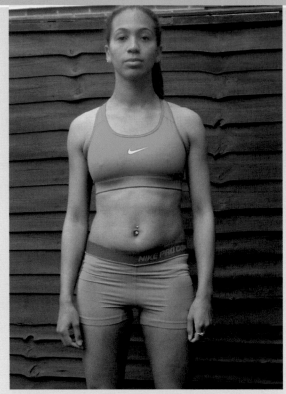

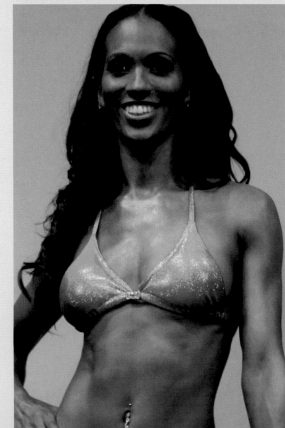

Natalie Jowett

TOTAL BODY TRANSFORMATION – THE RESISTANCE WAY

Natalie Jowett dramatically changed her body shape in the gym by taking on the challenge of using weights to sculpt a fitness model body.

'I had been one of the UK's top sprinters as an under-20 athlete but a persistent hip injury while at university meant I had to retire before reaching my prime. I was unable to train for the best part of four years and my motivation hit rock bottom. I continued to go to the gym but with nothing to train for my motivation to stay in shape waned.

'A few people suggested I should consider training for a show, but I dismissed the idea. Either way, I decided I needed a proper training programme to give my training some structure. I contacted a successful bodybuilder who trained at the gym and asked her for some advice on training and diet. She helped me to recapture my love of training and I started to enjoy going to the gym again and being in an environment where so many people were into bodybuilding and were passionate about training. Within a few months my progress was really marked and I loved the changes the training was making to my body. It seemed fitting then to start considering the possibility of competing.

'Having something to aim for helped maintain my focus and seeing the further improvement in my shape, condition, symmetry and overall body tone kept me motivated throughout the preparation. The diet was by far the most challenging thing I have ever done. The new diet consisted of eating every three hours and I really struggled at first. But after a couple of months I started to get used to it and found that I would start to get hungry after a few hours, whereas previously I could easily go for half of the day without eating.

'Throughout my show preparation my weight did not change a huge amount due to trading fat for muscle but my shape altered quite dramatically, especially in the final few weeks. On the day of the show I thought I would be nervous but surprisingly I wasn't, I just felt excited to get up on stage and felt confident because I was in the best shape of my life! I looked so different. I actually placed fourth and narrowly missed out on a place at the British Championship. I have had lots of positive feedback about my physique since the show and this has really spurred me on to compete again.'

Find out more about Natalie on Facebook

◀ Left: Natalie Jowett, before and after.

RESISTANCE TRAINING TERMINOLOGY

REPS: The number of lifts or movements of an exercise, be it body weight, suspension trainer, free or fixed weights.

SETS: The number of times a designated number of reps is repeated.

RECOVERY: The time taken betweens sets before repeating a set or moving on to the next exercise.

WEIGHT TO LIFT (ALSO KNOWN AS LOAD/RESISTANCE): Determined by the strength type aimed at and normally an actual or estimated percentage of 1 repetition maximum (one rep max/1RM). For suspension training and body weight exercises, resistance can be varied – for example, by adjusting the angle used to perform the exercise.

In the workout chapters (4 and 5), you'll find suggestions as to the weight to lift based on the terminology *light*, *light*/*medium*, *medium*, *medium*/*heavy* and *heavy*. You will find more information in these chapters.

TRAINING SYSTEM: The way the reps, sets and weight to lift are combined to produce a desired training outcome (see Table 4, page 41).

LIFTING SPEED: Resistance exercises have a concentric and eccentric phase (with weights, these apply to the lifting and lowering phases respectively). Varying the speed of these two components of a lift can influence the outcome of a workout or training phase. For example, emphasising the eccentric phase, perhaps by using a 5–10 second 'lower' count, can target greater numbers of fast twitch muscle fibres.

ONE REP MAX: As indicated, the maximum amount you could lift only once in a given exercise, or percentage of 1RM. You can also have a 6 reps max, an 8 reps max and so on, i.e. a weight that you could only lift 6 or 8 times respectively in one go. See page 28 for a reminder of ways to calculate your 1RM or rep maxes.

Resistance training systems

The way that reps, sets, recovery periods, resistance used and lifting speeds are combined will determine the training system that's used. Think of a training system as a recipe that binds all the training ingredients together. Training systems have different outcomes – for example, they may be better suited to developing one or a combination of the different strength types. This means that when specifically chosen and combined in a periodised training plan (see Chapters 4 and 5) you'll have the best opportunity to get the result you want from your training. Many of the systems described in Table 5 are used in the two 12-week programmes in Chapters 4 and 5. It's a good idea to familiarise yourself with these now. I hope that, by the end of this book, not only will you be in great shape but you will also be very confident when it comes to designing your own training programmes and working out what systems and exercises work best for you (and ultimately understand and use ones that are not contained in the programmes). Training progression requires consistency and variation. This may sound contradictory – you *do* need to repeat workouts but at the same time you don't want to let your mind and muscles get so used to them that they fail to respond and make positive physical changes. It's the aim of the 24-week programmes to achieve this.

Think of a training system as a recipe that binds all the training ingredients together

Weight Training Systems

TABLE 5

WEIGHT TRAINING SYSTEMS	DESCRIPTION	EFFECTS	COMMENTS
Simple sets (SS)	• Combines the same number of reps, e.g. 20 with a designated number of sets. Example: 4 x 20 at 50% 1RM	• Depends on the reps and percentage of 1RM used. For example, 4 x 20 reps at 50% of 1RM, with 30sec between sets, would develop strength endurance, while 4 x 3 reps at 85% 1RM would develop maximum strength.	• Despite their name, simple sets are a very effective way to resistance train – they are suitable for all levels of fitness. • You can vary the weight lifted, the number of reps and recovery to create different training outcomes.
Drop sets (DS)	• This intense method of training begins with a heavy load on the bar (for example, 75% plus 1RM). As many reps are completed as possible. Weight is then taken off the bar and as many reps as possible are completed again. This process continues for a designated number of sets or until there is no weight left on the bar! • Can also be done with dumbbells.	• This system will have a serious anabolic (growth) effect and significantly overload muscles (all fibre types). As such, it is a good option for increasing lean muscle mass and, potentially, size.	• This is an advanced system and should only be used very selectively by the suitably experienced. At least 48 hours' recovery must be taken after such workouts. Protein should be consumed immediately afterwards to help rebuild muscles (see Chapter 7).

| **Supersets (SuS)** | • Supersets contain pairings of exercises (or more – although these are usually called 'Giant sets', see below). The pairs can target the same muscle/muscle group – for example, the bench press and chest flyes for the pectorals. They can also work opposing muscle groups, such as the biceps and triceps, with biceps curls and triceps curls respectively. There are numerous other types of supersets. However, there is consistency with the way they are performed: one set is performed of one of the exercises in the pair, then the other immediately afterwards. A recovery is then taken between each pair before the next superset is performed. A type of superset can also be performed with a mix of weight training and plyometric (jumping) exercises that work the same muscle groups – for example, the squat and squat jump. This is also known as 'complex training'. Such training is great for boosting sports performance as it targets fast twitch muscle fibres. | • Supersets are great at hitting muscle fibre and stimulating growth, particularly if they target the same muscle group and medium to heavy weights are used.
• The training programmes in Chapters 4 and 5 use supersets and the pairings are designed to balance strength development across muscle groups and actions, and build metabolically active lean muscle. | • Suitable for all intermediate and advanced weight trainers.
• Complex training will benefit your sport's performance if you play tennis, football, netball or similar. |
| **Giant sets (GS)** | • Giant sets are similar to supersets – they involve any number of sets of exercises performed one after the other with recovery between each giant set. | • Giant sets can, for example, focus on a specific body part/area or use exercises that utilise different muscular actions or they can just be a random grouping of exercises. | • An intermediate/advanced option. Due to their intensity, giant sets can be very useful for building lean muscle as they can create a very positive hormonal response. To do this, it is best to use a medium/medium to heavy weight. |

Pyramids (P)	• Pyramids can increase or decrease in terms of the percentage of 1RM used on each set – that is, each set can use more or less weight and more or less reps, depending on whether the pyramid is an escalating or descending one.	• Most pyramids enable you to tackle heavier and heavier weights with a staggered approach (the increasing pyramid). For example: 1 x 8 at 75% 1RM 1 x 6 at 85% 1RM 2 x 4 at 90% 1RM	• An intermediate/ advanced option.
Split routine (SR)	• Specific body parts, such as the legs, chest and shoulders, are exercised in separate workouts over a training period (usually a week). This enables maximum effort to be put into training a specific body part on each day, e.g. legs on Monday, chest on Wednesday, shoulders on Friday.	• Great for those looking for increased muscle size and lean mass development – maximum mental and physical effort can be put into training each body part and the system allows for relatively long periods of muscle-growing recovery between workouts that target the same muscles.	• Suitable for intermediate and advanced trainers and those looking to increase muscle size.
Negative (eccentric) lifts (NL)	• These workouts emphasise the lowering (eccentric muscular action) phase of the lift by lowering the weight to a slow 5–10 count. **Note**: super-maximum weights (100–120% plus of 1RM) achieve the best results. You will need a training partner and/or specifically adapted weight training/Smith machine training equipment to perform these workouts.	• Great for increased size, power and strength. Due to their capacity to target fast twitch muscle fibres, negatives are often used by power athletes (sprinters, footballers) in a training programme designed to develop maximum (and useable) strength that will benefit sports performance. • The inclusion of negatives in a training programme can have a positive effect on increasing concentric strength.	• Suitable for advanced trainers.
Forced reps (FR)	• With the aid of a training partner, you 'force' out 1 or 2 additional reps when you would not normally be able to do so at the end of your set/sets. These are commonly referred to as the 'growth reps'.	• This training system pushes your muscles into unknown territory, optimising the conditions for muscle growth.	• Advanced training option that requires considerable mental input. It should be used sparingly. Ensure sufficient recovery after these workouts. • A tough system suited to intermediate and advanced trainers. Suitable for all body types.

Escalating density training (EDT)	• A less-used training programme – you complete as many reps as you can of an exercise in a set time span – for example, as many press-ups as you can perform in 15min – and then try to beat that during subsequent workouts.	• Local muscular endurance predominately, with high metabolic cost.	• Pace judgement and mental toughness are key. You must select an appropriate weight (where relevant) and perform reps in a distributed way that will enable you to keep going for the time span. Not suited to beginners or those new to resistance training.
German volume training (GVT)	• This system uses a specific protocol, usually 10 x 10 reps, with a resistance of around 70% 1RM and very short recoveries – for example, 1min.	• Used by those wanting to increase lean muscle, a result of the high level of muscle-building hormones released as a response to the workout.	• An advanced method, requiring considerable mental effort. This system will likely produce muscular soreness and should be used sparingly in a training programme.
Circuit training (CT)	• Uses body weight exercises such as sit-ups and squats. High numbers of reps and sets and recoveries are normally short.	• Great for developing local muscular endurance and base condition.	• Great starting point for anyone commencing a resistance/sports or specific resistance training programme.
Circuit resistance training (CRT)	• Similar to CT, but uses moderate-weight resistance exercises. Could also include suspension trainer and plyometric exercises.	• As above, but will also develop increased power. Mainly targets slow twitch muscle fibre and can improve CV fitness too.	• As above, good base for a resistance training programme.
As many reps as possible (AMRAP)	• The idea is simply to complete as many reps as possible of a given exercise (usually using a low to medium weight) in a set period of time.	• Another method primarily for developing muscular endurance.	• Requires mental toughness – suitable for advanced trainers.

Please note that the abbreviations of these training systems are used in the training programmes you'll follow in Chapters 4, 5 and 6.

Training variables

Training variables, such as quantity, quality, load, intensity, duration, frequency and rest/recovery, are fundamental to constructing a progressive training plan – they inform and shape individual workouts, the training systems used and their outcomes. It's good to have an understanding of these, for greater ease of understanding of the workouts in Chapters 4, 5 and 6 and should you wish to construct your own training programmes in future.

QUANTITY

Quantity refers to the amount of training done, whether in a particular workout or as part of a particular training phase. It can be measured by the total weight lifted, repetitions or sets completed in the weights room or the number of jumps and ground contacts during a plyometric workout, for example.

QUALITY

Quality usually reflects the intensity of a workout. For weight training, the amount of recovery allowed between repetitions and sets and the speed of lifting reflect quality, so the longer the recovery the greater the quality, as this will enable more powerful lifting, less affected by fatigue.

LOAD

Specifically, load references the resistance that has to be overcome – it's most applicable to weights sessions but also applies to, for example, vibration training (where the load is measured by the vibration frequency and amplitude of the machine or suspension training where body angle and strap length can increase or decrease resistance).

INTENSITY

Load can also be used on a more general basis to reference the intensity of the training cycle. Shorter training phases, lasting usually a week to 10 days, should be progressed through light, medium and heavy load workouts, in order to create conditions for progressive adaptation. Failure to factor in sufficient recovery (within sessions and the overall training plan) will compromise training progression.

DURATION

Duration is normally applied to the length of a training session on the more general level or on a much more focused level to the lifting and lowering phases of a weights exercise (speed of lift) or time of hold for an isometric muscular action.

FREQUENCY

Frequency refers to the number of times you train over a week, a month or other designated time span or perform a certain type of workout.

REST/RECOVERY

Recovery (or rest) applies to the gaps between reps and sets. Recovery can be applied to the gaps between training sessions and training phases. These should include designated recovery periods (days). Without their inclusion, optimum adaptation to training will not happen.

SLEEP TO GET LEANER

You should aim for 7–8 hours of quality sleep each night. It's when you sleep that your mind, body and muscles recover, repair and regenerate. Hormonal activity continues overnight and much research exists pointing to optimized levels of release with 'good' sleep.

▶ What kit do you need?

You probably already have the majority of the kit you'll need for resistance training. Leggings (short or long) and a vest/T-shirt and track-top will do for most occasions. Normal running trainers will be OK to use when getting started but as you progress you'll benefit from more stable shoes – those with lower midsoles. This will apply when lifting heavier weights. Why? If you were squatting with a heavy bar on your shoulders or dumbbells held at arms' length, for example, then your body weight and the added weight will all be channelling through your feet to the ground through your shoes. If the midsole is high and squidgy, your base of support will be unstable and your ankles may roll outward or inward, which could lead to injury or the stressing of joints unnecessarily. This would be even more pronounced on single leg and more dynamic exercises, such as lunges. Hence it's better to use shoes with a relatively firm midsole that is lower to the ground. Cross trainers, or certain tennis shoes, make for good choices.

OTHER EQUIPMENT ADVICE

▶ Plyometric jumping-type exercises are best performed on a giving surface such as a sprung floor or gymnastics mat. More cushioned shoes are also a good choice. Suitable surfaces include gym mats, sprung floors and dry, flat grass.

▶ Weight training gloves are a sensible option when tackling dumbbells and barbells, to protect your hands.

▶ Weight training belts – it's better to learn proper technique, to strengthen your core through relevant exercises and to use intra-abdominal pressure (see page 47) as a brace for your core when lifting weights, than use a belt. Research indicates that they do not offer as much support as often thought and can also lull the wearer into a false sense of security/safety. Learning proper technique for an exercise is key and a belt is no substitute for this.

▶ Compression clothing – this is produced by the major gym kit makers as a means to protect and keep

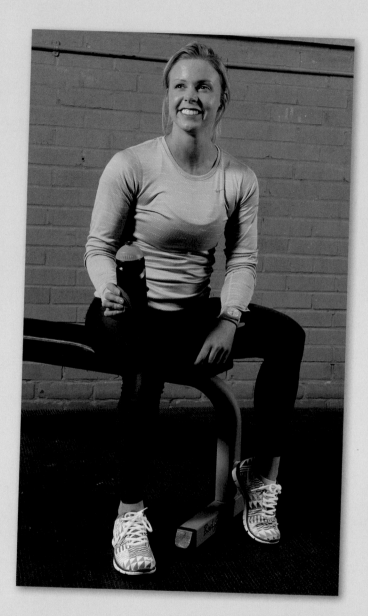

muscles warm. Some research indicates that it can be useful as the fit makes the wearer more aware of the muscles and their movements. Incidentally, compression clothing probably has greater claims as a means to boost recovery. If you think your muscles will be sore, you can wear compression clothing post workout or even while sleeping.

▶ Compound and isolation exercises

Compound exercises work multiple muscles across numerous joints – for example, the squat and lunge. Because of this, they require more physical and mental energy to perform and have a greater metabolic cost and hormone boosting effect.

Isolation exercises work smaller amounts of muscle across one joint – for example, the elbow and biceps when performing a biceps curl. They have much less of a metabolic and positive hormonal response.

As I stress throughout this book, muscle is metabolically active 24/7 and the leaner you are, the better calorie burner your body will be.

You will have more chance of creating a very efficient calorie burning body – one that burns fat each and every day – if you use compound exercises as opposed to isolation ones.

INTRA-ABDOMINAL PRESSURE (IAP)

The most effective way to brace your core when lifting, in order to protect it from injury, is through what is known as intra-abdominal pressure.

To create IAP, ready yourself as if you were about to be punched in the abdomen. Don't pull your naval inwards but rather tense your abdominals to fill your rib cage and sides. At the same time, squeeze and tighten your pelvic floor (as if you were trying to stop the flow of urine). At the same time, take a short intake of breath.

Certain lifts and positions when performing a weights exercise will particularly benefit from IAP – for example, during a step up onto and down from the step.

HOW MANY TIMES A WEEK DO I TRAIN?

To reiterate, it's in the time when you are not training that the positive adaptations to your workouts take place, i.e. when your muscles get stronger (more powerful or more enduring, depending on desired strength outcomes) and you increase functional capacity and leanness. It's sometimes easy to think that 'more is better' when it comes to working out, especially if you are new to training (and have just set your New Year's resolutions!). However, doing too much (for example, too many workouts or sessions that are too intense, too soon) can lead to compromised adaptation, as your muscles don't have sufficient time to recover, leading to increased tiredness and, at worst, injury. The programmes that follow in Chapters 4 and 5 allow for rest, in terms of easy and hard weeks of training and specific rest days. Nutrition (see Chapter 7) is also crucial in terms of optimising recovery and adaptation, as is quality sleep.

4 PATH TO RESISTANCE 1

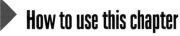 Training programme: Weeks 1 to 12

You want flat abs, no bingo wings, a pert bottom, a flat, toned stomach and slender, cellulite-free legs. So where do you start? Well, you resistance train! In this chapter you'll find a 12-week training plan that will put you well on your way to building the body of your dreams (in Chapter 5, you'll find a more advanced programme over a further 12 weeks that'll take your fitness and body to the next level). You'll also find plenty more positive and motivating comment from women who have trodden the resistance training path and are living proof of the resistance way.

▶ How to use this chapter

In this chapter you'll find the exercises that you'll be doing, with photographs and descriptions, followed by the workout programme. The first 6-week period primarily uses body weight exercises to start your resistance training journey, although some dumbbell variants are included. This means that you could do your workouts at home. The second half of the first phase introduces more and heavier resistance exercises. It is possible to do most of these workouts at home too, although you may need to invest in some training equipment – for example, barbells, dumbbells or Powerbags.

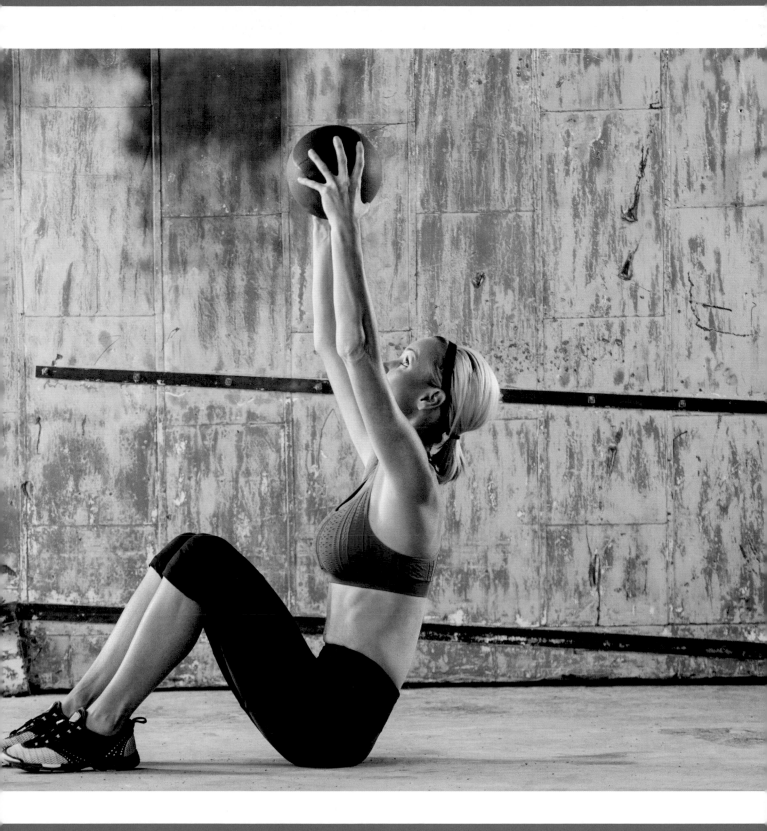

▶ What are Powerbags?

Powerbags are soft, cylindrical bags normally filled with sand. They have two grips and come in sizes from 3kg to 50kg plus (6.5lb to 110lb). The majority of barbell exercises described in this book could be performed using a powerbag. As they are relatively safe to drop, they are suited to home use. One version can be filled with sand and water across a number of compartments, offering a variable resistance of between 6kg and 25kg (13–55lb).

The workouts in the week-by-week tables contain the training system to use (see Chapter 3, p41-44) and the suggested reps and sets and rest periods as well as the exercises. I recommend that you spend time reading through the exercise descriptions and also try any that you are unsure of, before going full blast into the workouts. This is especially important if you have little or no exercise experience or have had a long layoff from relevant training. (Note: where there is a significant change in workout emphasis, workouts are often introduced in the transition week that focus on learning the correct technique for the key new exercises).

▶ Have a think

You should consider your strengths and weaknesses and any injury concerns, training history and your age. The 'right' resistance exercises will strengthen your body and improve both function and form, but choosing the 'wrong' ones or not adhering to good technique could lead to injury. If you are in any doubt about your suitability for exercise, do consult your doctor or a fitness professional.

▶ Anita Coleman

SIZE 18 TO 8: THE RESISTANCE TRAINING WAY!

Anita Coleman is a single mother of two beautiful children (a boy and a girl) and an inspiration to many women (and men). She trains hard and eats as healthily as she can. With thousands of social media followers she's motivating so many others and shows, that as a single mum, you can find the time to live a fit and healthy lifestyle.

▶ A fit family

Anita explains that she runs a fit family. 'We are a very active family. Health and fitness is a big "yes" in our family and we love being active and eating healthy.'

Anita was into sport and exercise in her school days – she played hockey and ran and was a keen horse rider. However, she let things slip as family life took hold. Her current interest in getting fit came after having her second child. Anita explained that with each pregnancy she put on five stone and went from a size 8 to a size 18 in nine months. 'After the first pregnancy the weight came off very easily, but with the second it was much more difficult. I lost the first three stone relatively easily but struggled with the last one to one and a half.' Anita was breastfeeding throughout. So to try to shift the remaining weight, she decided to do a sponsored three-mile fun run for Sport Relief. She went out four nights a week to train and the remaining weight did come off. However, as Anita puts it, she was 'left with a saggy stomach and loose skin'. In an attempt to tackle this, she went to her local gym, but as she readily admits she didn't have a clue as to what to do. She explained that the gym staff were very helpful and got her lifting weights. 'I will admit that I was thinking "I don't want to get 'manly'"', as back then I was not very educated about health and fitness and thought I might build unattractive muscle. But I trusted what they said and within seven weeks I was seeing results and I was getting more into it.'

▶ Motivation

Like many people, motivation – finding it and keeping it – is crucial to Anita when it comes to maintaining her size eight figure. She explains that to keep working out and following a healthy diet, she takes progress photos of herself. 'I take one every week to see if there is any change.' She often posts these on her Instagram page. She explains that she finds healthy eating easier to adhere to. 'I eat pretty healthy and clean all year round.' In terms of advice for other women (and men) wanting to get and stay in shape, she advocates plenty of rest between workouts and proper nutrition: 'If you don't rest properly or eat sensibly you can get easily fatigued and lose motivation.'

'Maintaining my physique and fitness can be hard work at times, especially being a single mum and working as well,' explains Anita, adding, 'It can be tiring and sometimes, especially when I have been at work all day and I'm stressed with everyday living, I can lose

motivation at times.' So how does she turn the negatives into a positive? 'But when I do feel like this I will think to myself and say, "Look how far you have come with transforming your body, keep going, don't give up now." And after lifting weights for five years now it has become an everyday routine for me.'

▼ Below: Anita Coleman.

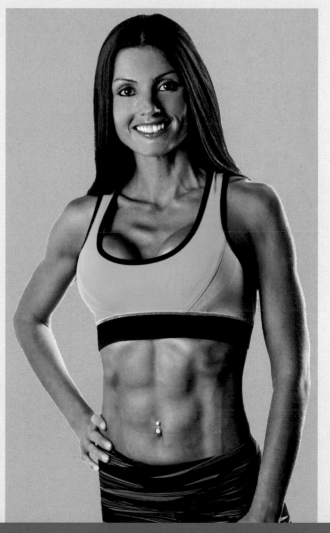

▶ Machine vs Free Weights

Free weights include kettlebells, dumbbells, barbells and Powerbags, for example. Weight machines are those normally designed with selector-based weight stacks. Some argue that the latter are safer and should be used by people new to weight training. However, this is not actually the case as, in some ways, machine weights can create as many problems as they are supposedly designed to overcome. Firstly, they are often constructed for the average-sized person (not even the average man or woman), so if you are taller or smaller, it can result in compromised body positions in the machine, which can stress joints unnecessarily. Secondly, machines can disconnect the muscles/movement targeted from the rest of the body. For example, a machine squat can only follow a fixed path as the machine controls the movement. Although your legs and glutes supply the power to lift and lower the weight, they do not have to stabilise the movement. This stabilisation uses a myriad of other muscles – working from your ankles to your neck. Consider this, too: if you were to squat down to sit in a chair, for example, you have to balance; if you reach to take an object from a shelf above you, you need balance and stability across the whole body. This is why free weights are preferable to fixed weight machines as they reflect how your muscles are used in 'real life' and therefore have far greater transference and relevance. This is what makes free weights much more functional – of which more later. The most important aspect when it comes to free weights is learning correct technique and progressing sensibly. Don't be put off by them!

▶ Functional exercise

Following on from the 'fixed versus free weights' debate, there's been a huge push recently towards 'functional exercise' in the fitness industry. As someone who has been writing about fitness, sport, training and coaching for over 20 years, I find this quite alarming, as shouldn't all exercise be functional? What's the point of training if the training you are doing is not going to improve your functional, everyday capacity, or sports performance? One of the key aspects of what makes an exercise functional is its ability to allow the body to work as it was designed to, i.e. synergistically. This means that its movements must be multi-planar – three-dimensional. Everyday movements require us to bend (forwards and backwards and sideways), rotate (clockwise and anticlockwise), and move forwards, backwards and sideways. Very often these patterns also require acceleration and deceleration, as is the case when you pick up an object off the floor – the speed of its movement increases and then slows to a stop when you have the object at the level where you want it. It's obvious, but there are an infinite number of options for the way we can move.

The exercises in the practical workout chapters of this book are all functional – whether using your body weight or involving free weights. They are designed to strengthen your muscles collectively and to use numerous movement patterns. They also require you to control your speed and adjust your balance and also target all muscle actions (see Chapter 3). Consequentially, they'll improve not only your body shape, lean muscle levels and therefore calorie burning, but also your functional movement capacity and your athleticism.

▶ The exercises

You'll find the exercises used in this chapter and the first 12 weeks of your programme over the following pages. They've been divided up, where practical, into lower, core, upper body and all-body exercises (specifically designed to engage leg, core and arms together), with added resistance exercises (predominantly barbell/dumbbell exercises). A note is made of the muscles they specifically target and on occasions the specific muscular action they use. Tips, comments and other benefits are also provided and, where relevant, adaptations to the exercise are described to assist your understanding of correct technique or to make the exercises either harder or easier to perform.

The aim of the programme in this chapter is to introduce you to body weight exercises and some key weight training exercises that you'll use throughout the programme, such as the squat and dead lift. Additionally you'll be training to get into the shape necessary to complete more dynamic all-body exercises.

MOVING ON

Chapter 5 progresses workouts even more; resistances are upped and more new exercises introduced – for example, using kettlebells. Ultimately this will lead to achieving greater functional fitness and fat burning capability. Chapter 5 also includes suspension trainer exercises. (Note: if you are familiar with these types of exercise, you could include them in the workouts outlined in this chapter. You could swap a like-for-like (or close match) exercise with a suspension trainer one – for example, suspension trainer squats for body weight squats or the suspension trainer atomic press-up for the Brazilian crunch.)

Chapter 6 introduces more exercises and systems, such as High Intensity Training, and considers CrossFit®. It is more of a stand-alone chapter with sample workouts. BOSU ('both sides up') exercises are also included, as are a selection of other exercises that you can do to take your training to the next level.

▼ Try press-ups using a suspension training system.

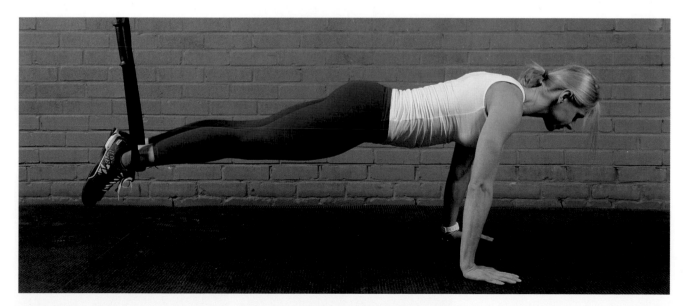

LOWER BODY EXERCISES

BODY WEIGHT

Squat

- Stand with your feet shoulder-width apart and look straight ahead.
- Hold your hands in front of you
- Bend your knees and lower until your thighs are approximately parallel to the floor (do not allow your heels to lift off the floor).
- Extend your legs to stand up, extending your hips as you do so. Maintain the natural curves of your spine. Keep your knees tracking over your feet.

TARGET MUSCLES AND FUNCTIONAL BENEFITS

- Calves
- Hamstrings
- Quads
- Glutes

Lower to a 2 count, lift to a 1 count

TIP

Next time you are sitting at home on your sofa, don't use your arms to aid getting up. Instead, slide your bottom near to the edge of the cushion, focus your energy and just use your legs.

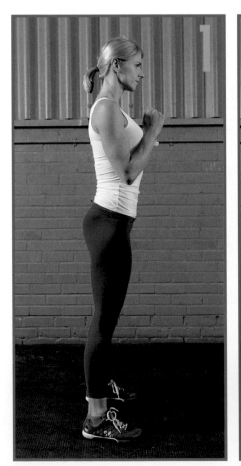
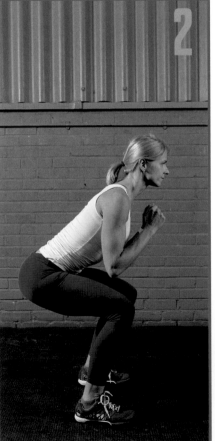

Single leg squat

- Stand with your arms held straight out in front and roughly parallel to the floor.
- Lift one leg to about a 45-degree angle in front of you.
- Focus and look straight ahead and then lower your bottom over your heel to squat down. Lower as far as your strength and balance allows. Do not allow your heel to lift off the floor. Complete all your reps on one leg and then repeat on the other.

Lower to a 2 count, lift to a 1 count

+|+TIP

Inclining your trunk forwards can allow you to squat lower. As with all squats, make sure your knee stays behind your toes when you lower and push up.

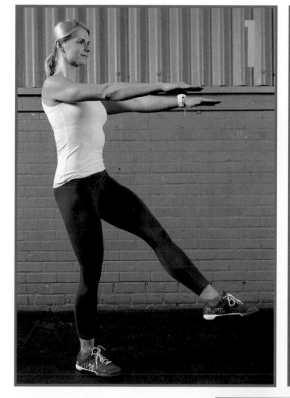

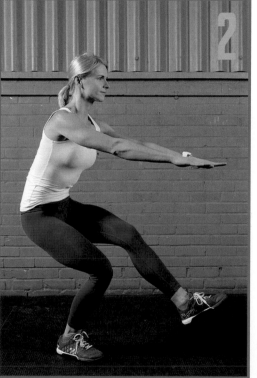

VARIATION
The exercise can also be performed with a low bench positioned behind you. This gives you a target to squat to – aim to lightly brush the bench with your bottom before pushing back up.

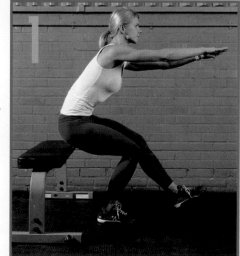

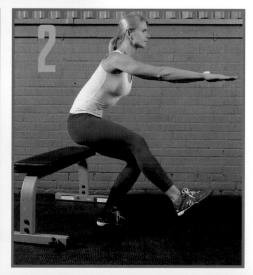

Squat into front kick

■ Stand with your feet shoulder-width apart and your hands held in front. Squat as described on page 54.

■ Next, and while maintaining the natural curves of your spine, lift out of the squat, kicking one leg up and out as you do so. Lead with the knee, before extending the leg.

■ Bring the kicking leg to the floor, pause and repeat, this time kicking the other leg out as you rise up from the squat.

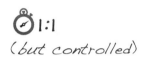

1:1
(but controlled)

TIP

Don't kick your leg out too vigorously – work within the limits of your strength and flexibility.

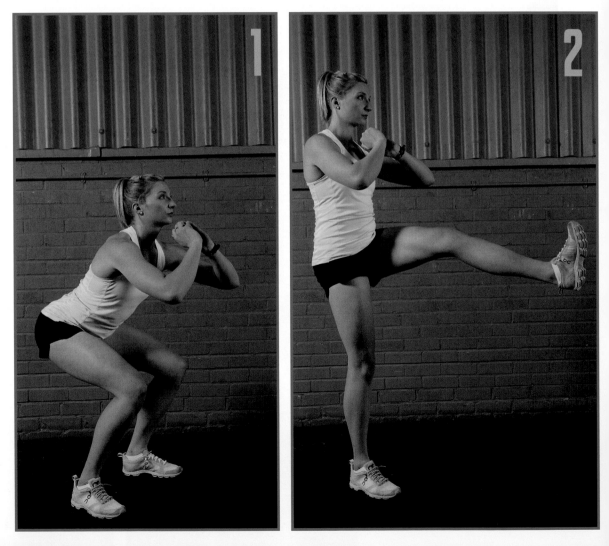

Squat into rear kick

■ Stand with your feet shoulder-width apart and hands held in front. Squat as described on page 54.

■ As you lift out of the squat, kick one leg out behind you, leading with your heel. You'll need to lean forward to do this.

■ Pull the leg back in and place the foot on the floor.

■ Reset and repeat, this time kicking out with your other leg.

Squat as described on page 54.

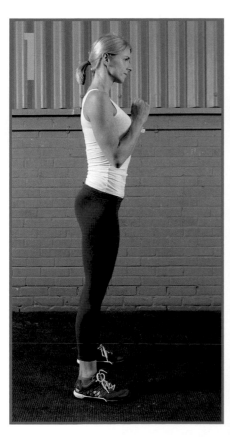

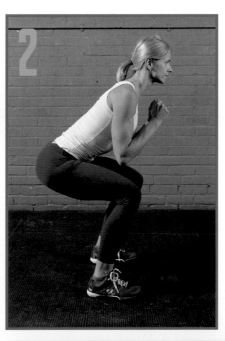

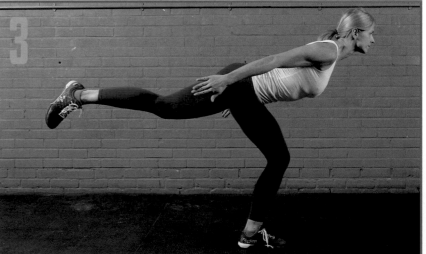

TARGET MUSCLES AND FUNCTIONAL BENEFITS

• Glutes
• Hamstrings
• Quads
• Hip flexors
• Calves
• Balance
• Body awareness
• Agility
• Flexibility

🕙 1:1
(but controlled)

⫞TIP

As with the previous exercise, perform with control.

Wall squat

- Place your hands by your sides.
- Position yourself against a sturdy wall so that your back is flat against it and your thighs are parallel to the floor, with your feet a shoulder-width apart.
- Hold this position for a set time. Try not to hold your breath.

TARGET MUSCLES AND FUNCTIONAL BENEFITS

- Glutes
- Quads
- Hamstrings
- Uses an isometric muscular action

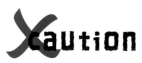

TIP

Make the exercise more difficult by consciously pushing back as hard as you can into the wall through your thighs.

Xcaution

This exercise should not be performed by those with high blood pressure.

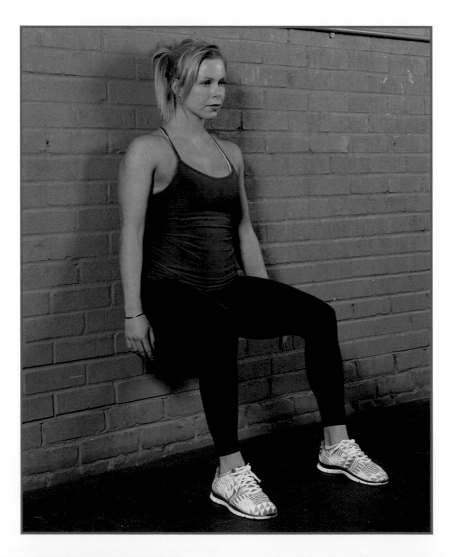

Squat into knee lift

- Stand tall with your hands by your ears and your elbows up. Squat down so that your thighs are parallel to the floor.
- As you lift out of the squat, lift one leg up and out to the side so the thigh is above parallel to the floor.
- Control the foot back to the floor, smoothly reset yourself with both feet on the floor and repeat, this time lifting the other leg as you lift out of the squat.

TARGET MUSCLES AND FUNCTIONAL BENEFITS

- Glutes
- Quads
- Hamstrings
- Calves
- Hip flexors
- Adductors and abductors
- Balance
- Flexibility

⏱ 1:1
(but controlled)

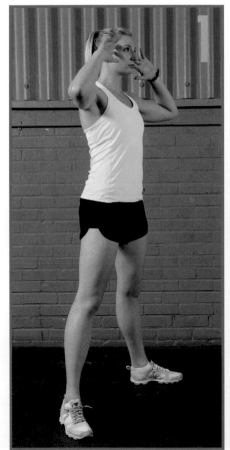
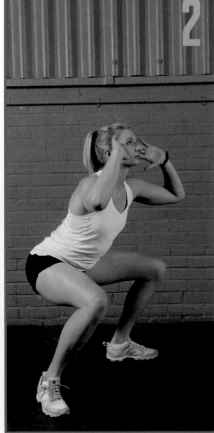
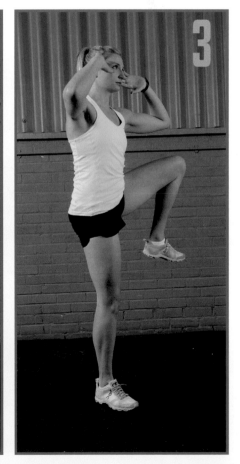

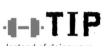 1:1
(but controlled)

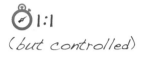TIP

Instead of doing your lunges in one spot, you can lunge forwards in a straight line. This is called a travelling/walking lunge. You can perform 10 or any even number of reps. Travelling lunges make for a great inclusion as an exercise in the Escalating Density Training system. Count up the number of lunges you complete and try to beat it next time. For a more detailed explanation of EDT training, see Chapter 3. Be warned, though – this is a tough workout!

Lunge

■ Stand with your hands by your sides.
■ Take a large step forwards into a lunge, keeping your chest elevated. Make sure the thigh of the lunging leg is near parallel to the floor and that your knee remains behind your toes. There should be a 90-degree angle at the knee of the rear leg.
■ Push through the heel of the lunging leg to return to the start position and take a large step forward to perform a lunge with the other leg.

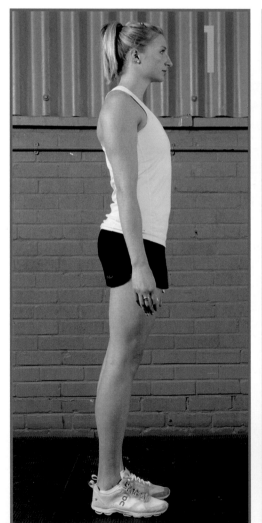

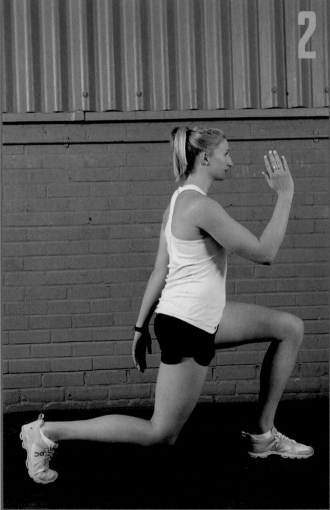

Side lunge

- Stand with your feet shoulder-width apart.
- Take a large step to one side to lunge sideways – you can bend your torso forwards as you do this.
- Bend the non-lunging leg to a position where the thigh is nearly parallel to the floor.
- Push back through the heel of the non-lunging leg and bring the lunging leg back to the start position.
- Reset and repeat with the other leg.

⏱ 1:1
(but controlled)

⊢⊩TIP

Don't try to lunge too far to the side. Keep the movement controlled and power up off the non-lunging leg when returning to the start position.

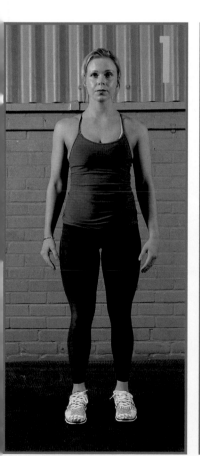
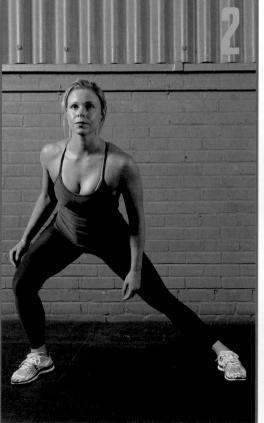
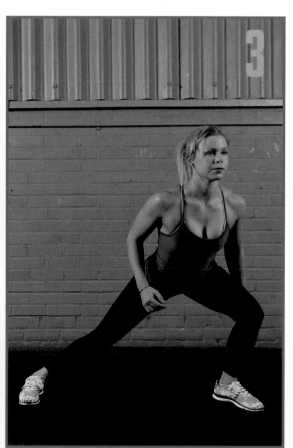

Curtsey lunge

- Stand and place your hands on your hips.
- Take a medium step forwards and outside the line of your back foot (i.e. across your body). Place your foot on the floor with toes facing forward.
- Bend your legs to squat.
- Push back through the heel of the lunging leg to return to the start position.
- Pause, then complete the exercise with the other leg leading.

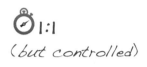 1:1
(but controlled)

TIP
Control the movement and keep your balance.

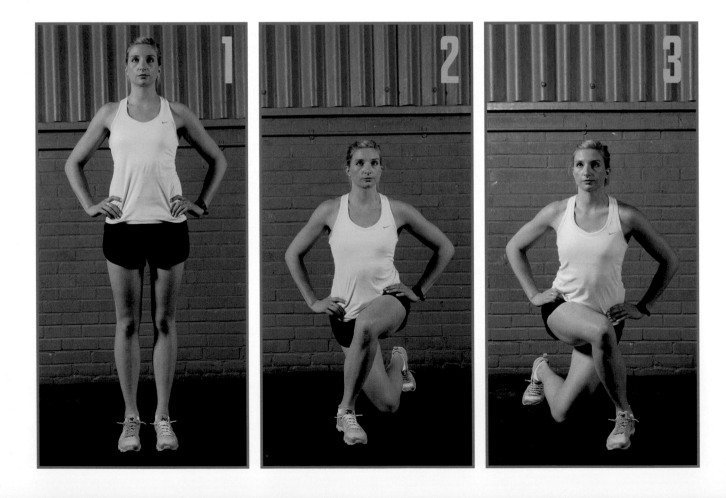

Speed skater

- Stand with your feet shoulder-width apart.
- Jump to your left to land on your left foot. As you do so, take your right leg behind the left.
- Immediately jump to the right and on landing take the left leg behind the right.

This is a high metabolic cost exercise that will increase your calorie burn!

⫶⊢ TIP

Keep to a steady pace. Lean slightly forwards throughout. Use your arms for balance and to add to your jump power. Make your landings light and quick.

🕐 1:1
(but controlled)

TARGET MUSCLES AND FUNCTIONAL BENEFITS

- Glutes
- Hamstrings
- Quads
- Adductors and adductors
- Calves
- Core
- Balance
- This is also a dynamic plyometric exercise

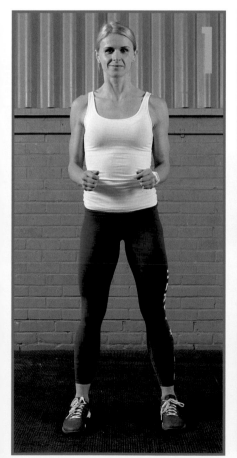
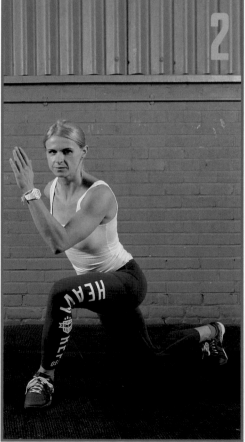
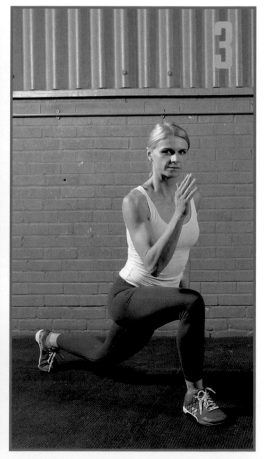

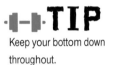

1:1
(but controlled)

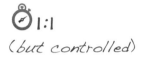

TIP

Keep your bottom down throughout.

Groiners

- Start in a press-up position.
- Jump one leg in, so that the foot lands beside your hand on the same side of your body.
- Jump the leg back and then switch legs. Continue alternating.

This is a high metabolic cost exercise that will increase your calorie burn!

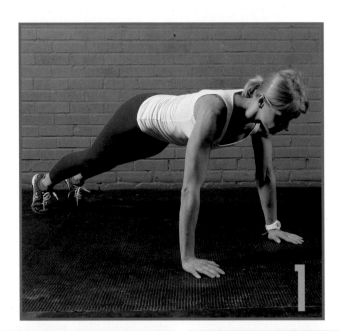

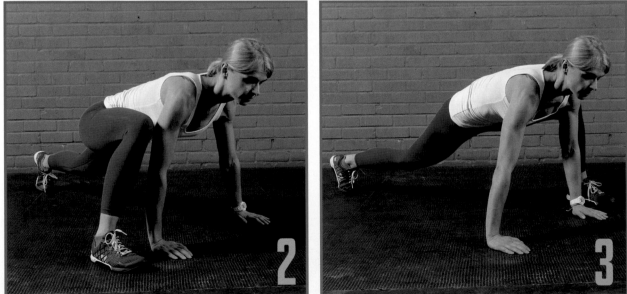

Glute bridge

- Lie on your back on the floor and place your hands by your sides.
- Bend your knees and lift your hips until there is a 90-degree angle at your knees (the bridge).
- Hold this bridge position and then lower under control.

 1:2

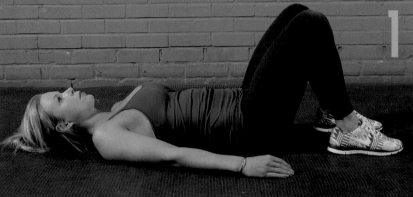

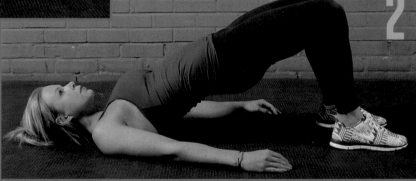

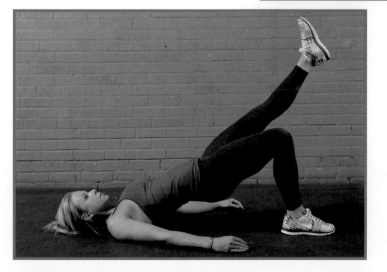

VARIATION

You can also lift one leg off the floor alternately from the elevated position. With this option, hold the thigh of the extended leg parallel to the thigh of the grounded leg.

Jump squat

■ Stand with your feet shoulder-width apart.

■ Bend your legs until your thighs are nearly parallel to the floor.

■ Dynamically extend your legs to leap into the air.

■ Land lightly and jump again

⏱ 1:1
(but controlled)

⫸ TIP

Use your arms to assist your jump power, by swinging them backwards and forwards in time with your jump. Land lightly, first on the balls of your feet before contacting the floor with your heels, and then power up into another jump.

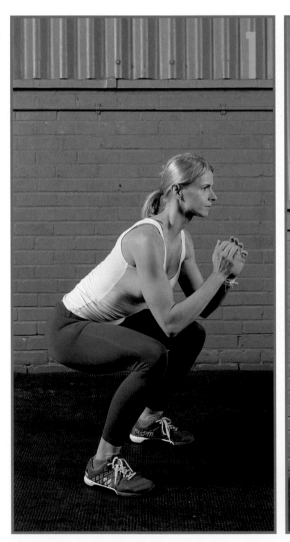

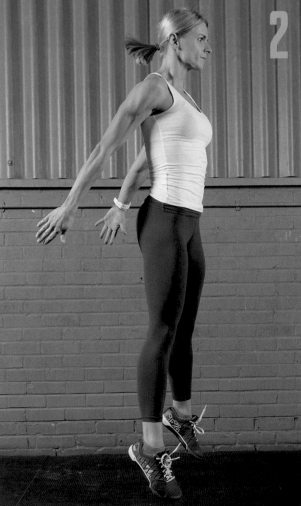

Plié jump

- Stand with your feet wider than shoulder-width apart and turned out. Make sure your feet and knees are angled similarly.
- Place your hands by your ears and keep your chest elevated.
- Bend your knees and then dynamically jump into the air, maintaining your foot spacing.
- Land lightly and then jump again.

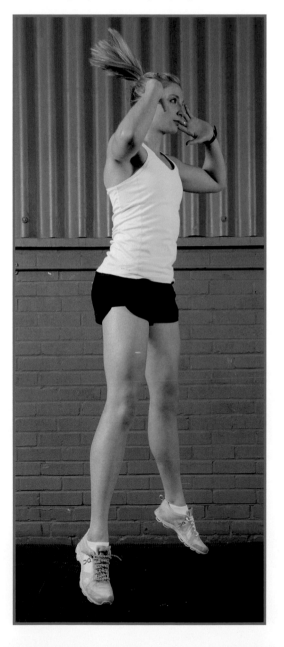

1:1
(but controlled)

TARGET MUSCLES AND FUNCTIONAL BENEFITS

- Glutes
- Adductors and abductors
- Hip flexors
- Hamstrings
- Calves
- This is also a plyometric exercise

WHY DO PLYOMETRIC EXERCISES?

Plyometric (jumping) exercises use a combination of muscle actions – specifically, an eccentric, lengthening one on landing from a jump followed immediately by a concentric, shortening one. Such a combination literally 'fires' your muscles to make you jump higher or move more quickly. This makes these exercises great for sports training (for netball, football, hockey and running and sprinting, for example). However, they are great for fitness training too as they have a high metabolic cost and are also fun. When you perform them, make sure you wear well-cushioned shoes and that you are jumping on a suitable surface – for example, dry flat grass, a running track, gym mat or sprung floor. If you are not used to jumping exercises, or have weak ankles and knees, for example, then reduce the volume of the exercises performed, or replace them with similar but non-plyometric alternatives – for example, the squat for the jump squat. When suitably conditioned, the key to their performance is speed of reaction to and off the floor. If you are in any way unsure about your suitability for performing these exercises, consult your doctor or suitable fitness professional.

CORE EXERCISES

Scissors

■ Lie on your back with your chin lifted and place your arms out to your sides, 20cm or so off the floor.
■ Keeping your legs straight, lift each leg up and back towards your head in a scissoring-type movement.

⏱ 1:1
(but controlled)

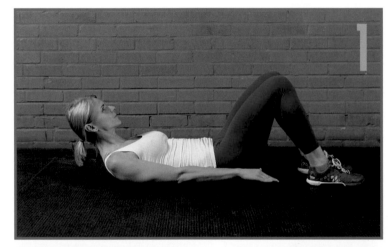

⊦⊢ TIP

Engage your core throughout. Work within the realms of your flexibility and don't swing the legs up – rather lift and lower with control. Really focus on combating gravity on each downward movement of the legs. Make sure you maintain the natural curves of your spine and don't 'force-arch/flatten' your back as you lift and lower.

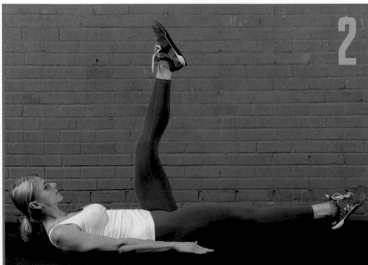

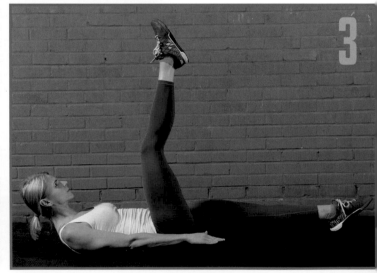

Russian twist

- Sit on the floor and lift your legs so they are bent to 90 degrees. Keep your torso up and your gaze straight ahead.
- Rotate your body from left to right, keeping the weight in place in front of your chest. You can also perform this exercise with your bodyweight by clasping your hands. Note that the movement is initiated from the torso and not through arm movement and momentum.

TARGET MUSCLES AND FUNCTIONAL BENEFITS

- Rectus abdominis
- Obliques
- Back
- Hip flexors

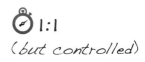 1:1
(but controlled)

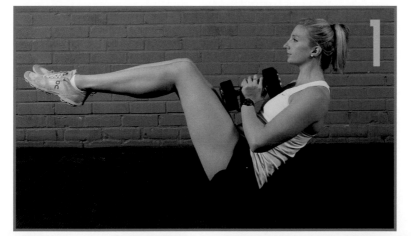

-|-|-TIP

You can perform the exercises with added resistance as pictured, using, for example, a dumbbell or medicine ball held centrally to your lower torso.

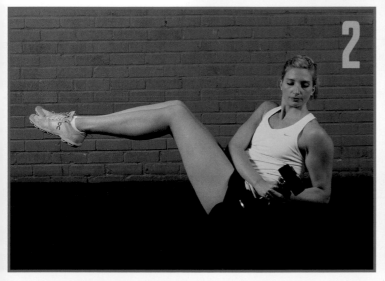

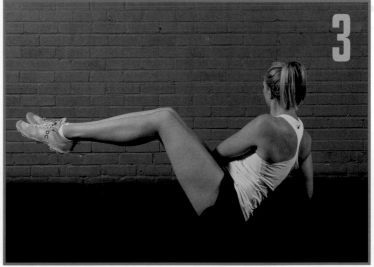

Feet elevated crunch

- Lie on your back with your hands by your sides.
- Lift your legs so they are close to vertical.
- Hold your legs in position as you 'crunch' your abdominals to lift your torso from the floor. Keep your arms parallel to the floor and lifted. Control the movement slowly up and down.

◄┠TIP

Don't swing your body up – engaging your abdominal muscles is key to developing great strength in your core.

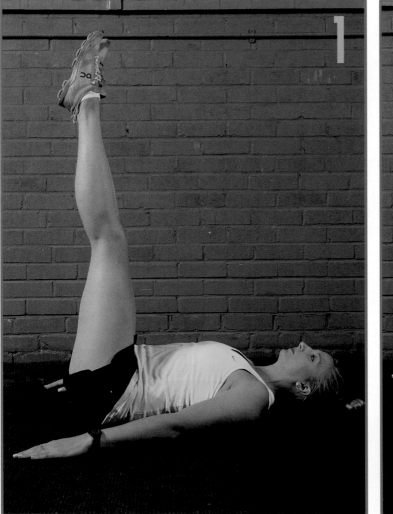

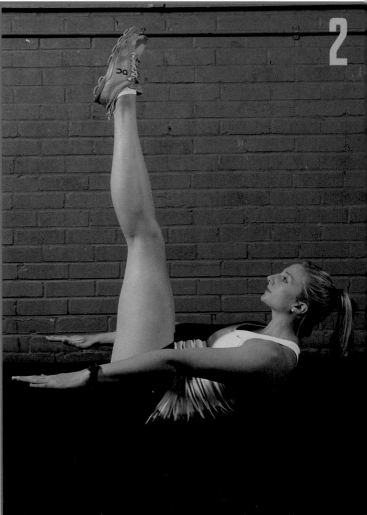

Reverse curl with toe touch

- Lie on your back with your hands by your sides and your legs in front of you, knees bent.
- Crunch your abs as you bend your legs to lift your lower back and legs from the floor.
- Slowly unfold your legs to tap the floor with your toes before transitioning into another rep (don't rest them on the floor).

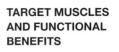 1:1
(but controlled)

This exercise is all about control and the constant tension in your core will make it more difficult than it seems.

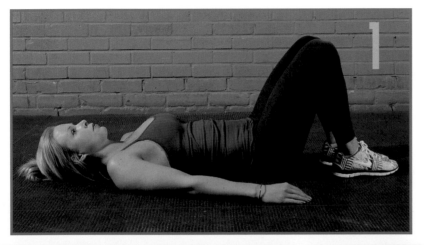

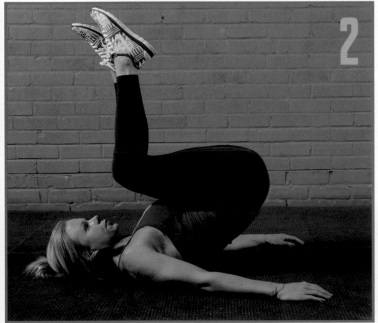

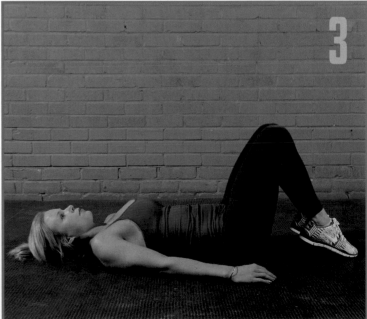

Straight arm plank

■ Assume a press-up position.
■ Support your body weight on your hands and toes, keeping the whole length of your body in a straight line. Don't sag, but maintain the natural curves of your spine – get a training partner or PT to 'line you up'.
■ Breathe throughout as you hold for a designated time span.

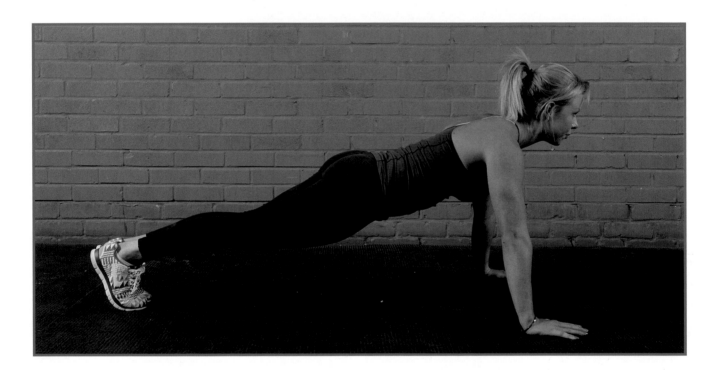

Plank

- Assume a prone position with your weight supported on your forearms and toes. As with the press-up plank, keep the whole length of your body in a straight line. Breathe throughout. Your abdominals should feel the pressure of holding your body still and your back should be engaged to offer further control.
- Hold for a dedicated time span.

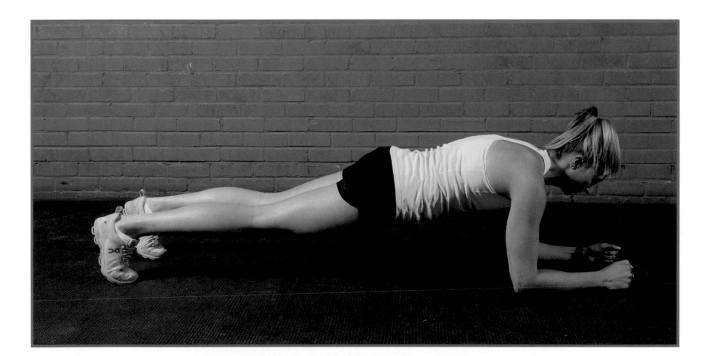

Plank and leg lift

■ Assume the same position as for the plank, but this time lift one leg to about a 45-degree angle, pause and then lower it. You can either alternate legs or complete a designated number of reps to one side before swapping over.

TARGET MUSCLES AND FUNCTIONAL BENEFITS

- Core (front, back and sides)
- Shoulders
- Glutes
- Hamstrings

🕑 1:2

⚡ TIP

With this exercise, it's important to keep your hips square to the floor and not to roll in and out as you lift and lower your legs.

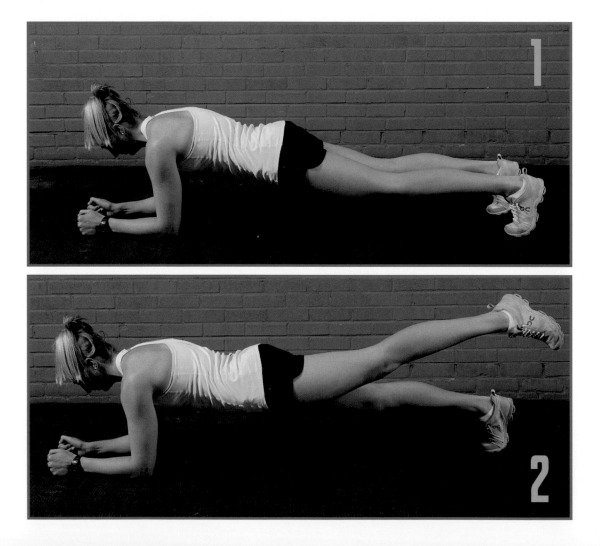

Reverse crunch

- Lie on your back with your knees bent, feet on the floor and arms by your sides.
- Squeeze your abs and lift your legs so that your lower torso, bottom and legs lift off the floor and move towards your head.
- Slowly unfurl to the start position. Lift only as far as your flexibility allows.

Lift only as far as your flexibility allows.

TARGET MUSCLES AND FUNCTIONAL BENEFITS

- Rectus abdominis

⏱ 1: 2

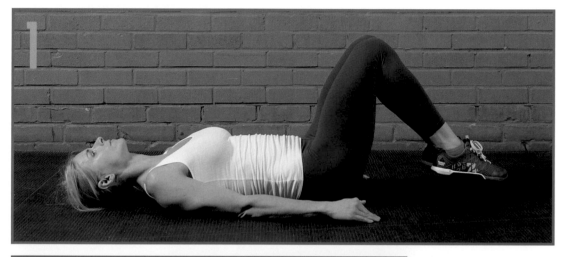

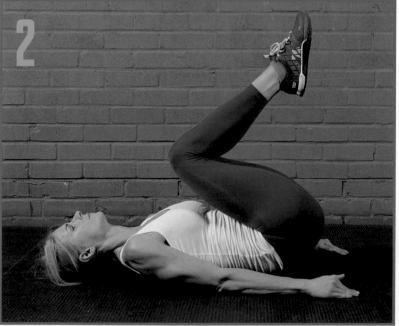

⊢ TIP

Make sure you squeeze with your abs. Don't swing your legs up – do this and you're cheating yourself and not getting the real benefit from the exercise. The slow approach also engages more muscle fibres and will therefore ultimately boost your body's metabolism and help you flatten your abdomen.

UPPER BODY EXERCISES

NOTE

Some of the exercises in the previous section, such as the Brazilian crunch, also work the chest and shoulders to a very high level.

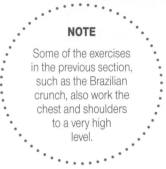

TARGET MUSCLES AND FUNCTIONAL BENEFITS

- Chest
- Shoulders
- Core

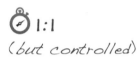

1:1
(but controlled)

Press-up

- Support yourself on your hands and toes, keeping your whole body in a straight line.
- Lower your chest towards the floor then extend your arms to push back up.

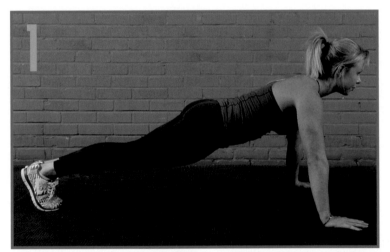

⊞— TIPS

- Perform press-ups from your knees for a slightly easier version.
- Altering your hand spacing will also change the emphasis of the exercise – for example, placing your hands below your shoulders puts more emphasis on your triceps.
- When performing a standard press-up, take your body to the floor in a straight line – don't lower your shoulders more than your torso or bottom. Do this and you'll perform the perfect press-up.

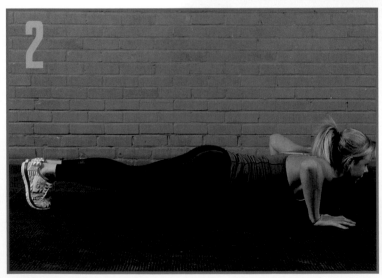

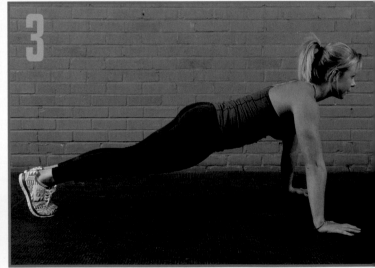

Triceps dips

- Sit on the floor.
- Support yourself on the flats of your feet and the palms of your hands and lift your hips to form a table-like position (your hands should be just behind your hips).
- Bend your arms to lower your bottom to the floor – don't use your legs to assist you.
- Extend your arms to return to the start position.

 1:1

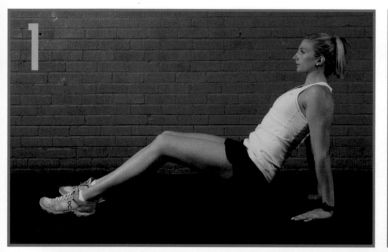

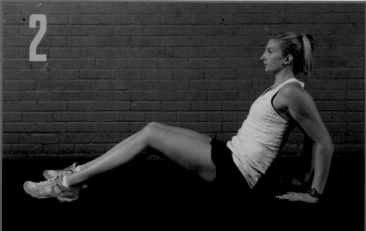

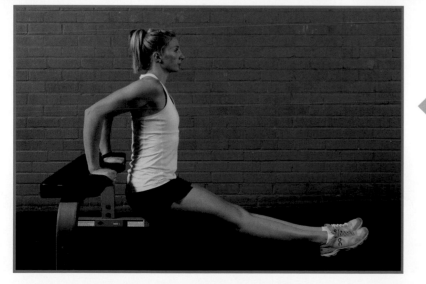

VARIATION

The exercise can also be performed using a chair (or similar object) by placing your hands on the edge of the seat. If doing the exercise this way, your legs can be bent for an easier option or extended for a harder one.

ALL-BODY EXERCISES

BODY WEIGHT

TARGET MUSCLES AND FUNCTIONAL BENEFITS

- Core
- Shoulders
- Chest
- Glutes
- Quads
- Calves

⏱ 1:1
(dynamic but controlled)

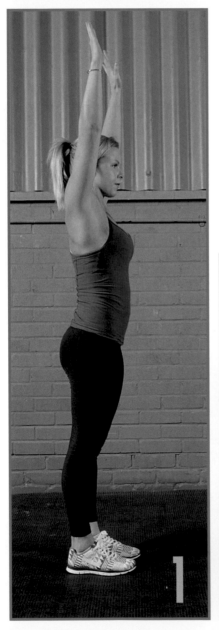

Burpee

- Stand, then bend your knees to place your hands flat on the floor and jump your legs back into a press-up position.
- Perform a press-up and then jump your legs back under your shoulders.
- As your feet strike the floor, jump up, lifting your arms overhead.
- Land lightly, bend your knees, put your hands back on the floor, jump your legs back and repeat.

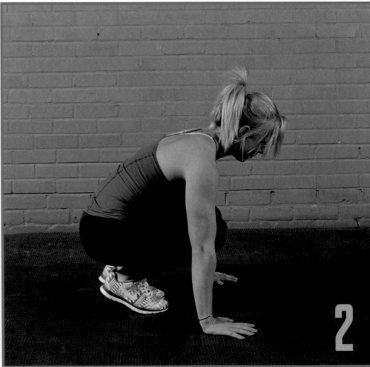

This is probably the toughest floor-based body weight exercise you can perform! The burpee works virtually every muscle in your body and has a very high metabolic cost – you could be out of breath after just a couple!

⊩TIP

If you find the exercise too tough to start with, omit the press-up and/or the jump part of the exercise, or break your reps down into chunks – i.e. if a set of 10 is prescribed, start with 4 and then take a short rest, do 3 and then a further 3.

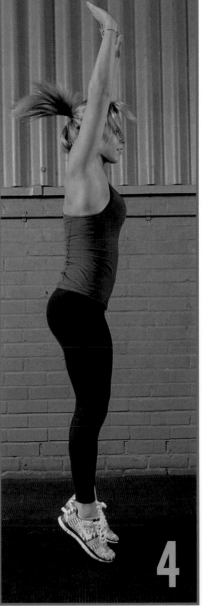

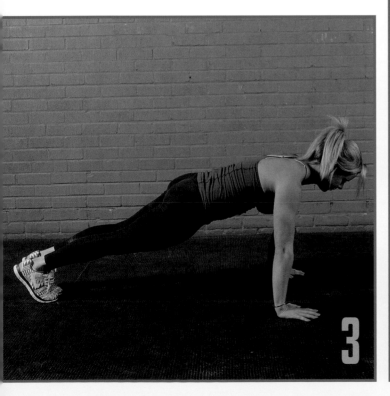

FREE WEIGHTS

As I mentioned earlier, this chapter also introduces you to selected key free weight exercises, such as the squat and dead lift, initially using relatively light weights. It's very important that you master the correct technique for these and other exercises before progressing to using heavier weights. You'll also find some new exercises, which can be performed with just body weight or with added resistance, e.g. dumbbells. There are also selected Swiss ball exercises, which often require you to engage your core more fully while performing an exercise, compared to similar floor-based exercises.

⏱ 1:1
(but controlled)

Rear foot elevated split squat

- Hold dumbbells at arms' length by your sides.
- Stand in front of a sturdy, suitable-height object e.g. a workout bench and place the toes of your rear foot on it.
- Hop your standing leg forward and place your foot flat on the floor.
- Keeping your trunk upright and looking straight ahead, bend your standing leg to lower your body until your thigh is approximately parallel to the floor.
- Push back up strongly and repeat. Avoid the temptation to assist the exercise with the rear leg.

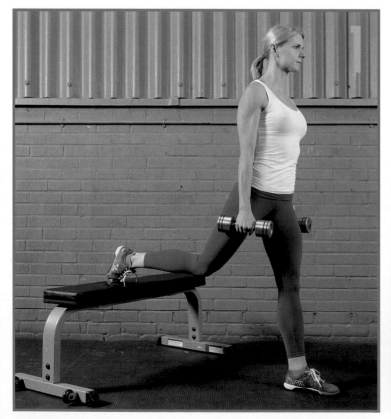

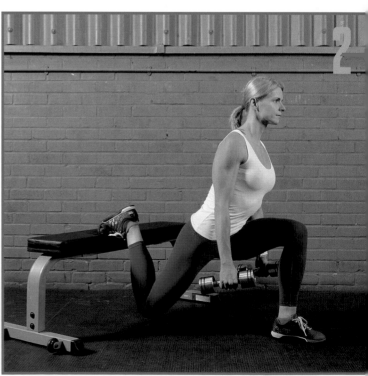

Swiss ball hamstring curl

- Lie on the floor and place your hands by your sides. Place your heels on top of the Swiss ball.
- Lift your hips so that your legs are straight.
- Keep pressing your heels into the ball as you pull the ball in towards you while maintaining the bridged position, and while you push it away. Get into a controlled rhythm.

TARGET MUSCLES AND FUNCTIONAL BENEFITS

- Glutes
- Hamstrings
- Core

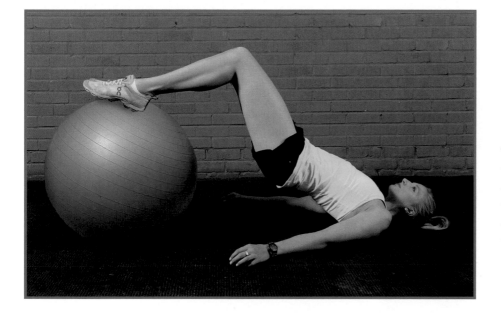

1:1
(but controlled)

TIP

You may need to reset yourself from time to time while performing a set. The more familiar you become with the exercise, the less this will happen. The exercise can also be performed one leg at a time and you can hold the bridge position to make it more of a plank-type of exercise.

training equipment

The right Swiss ball

Ensure that:

1 It's burst-resistant to a minimum of 500kg (1,100lb).
2 It meets British or international standards.
3 It is correct for your size.

Your Height (cm)	Ball size (cm)
152–168	55
168–188	65
188 plus	75

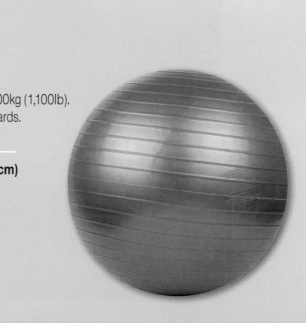

Reverse lunge with triceps extension

- Stand with your feet hip-width apart, holding the dumbbells in front of your chest with the heels of your hands pointing down.
- Take a large step backwards into a lunge by pushing back from the standing leg and lifting the other leg, up, back and down to place your toes on the floor. As you do so, extend your arms to perform the triceps extension.
- Step the rear leg back to the front while bringing the dumbbells back in to the starting position.
- Lunge back with the other leg, again performing the triceps extension.

1:1
(but controlled)

TARGET MUSCLES AND FUNCTIONAL BENEFITS

- Rear shoulders
- Back
- Triceps
- Glutes
- Quads
- Hamstrings
- Calves

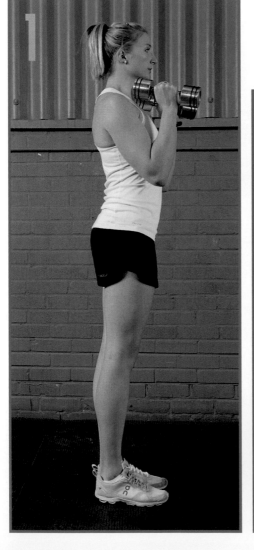

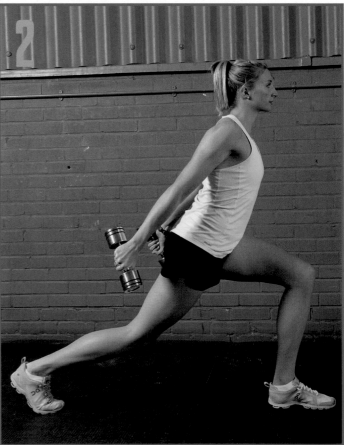

Single leg biceps curl to press

This is a great all-body exercise – you'll work numerous stabiliser muscles, too, while you hold position to move the weight using the prime movers, the arms and shoulders. A great deal of balance is also required as you hold yourself in place.

- Hold the dumbbells at arms' length by your sides with your knuckles down.
- Stand on one leg and lift the other leg until the thigh is parallel to the floor (you must hold this base position strongly throughout the exercise).
- Curl the weights up to your shoulders (don't swing them). Hold for a split second then rotate your wrists while at the same time pressing the weights to overhead, to perform the shoulder press part of the movement.
- Lower the weights under control and back to the start position, rotating your wrists at your shoulders to get the dumbbells positioned for the curl part of the next rep.

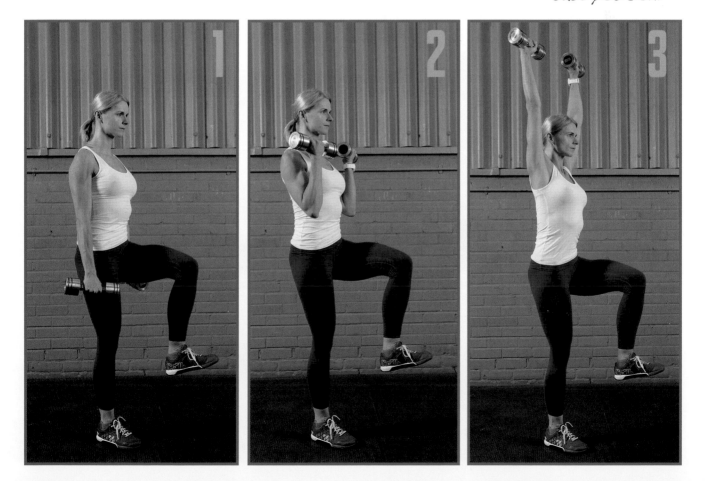

TARGET MUSCLES AND FUNCTIONAL BENEFITS

- In standing leg: Calf
- Hamstring
- Glutes
- In held leg: Hip flexor
- Core
- Biceps
- Shoulders

⏱ 1:1
(but controlled while holding the base position)

Lunge with weight held overhead

- Take hold of a weight's plate/dumbbell and hold it overhead with your arms straight.
- Take a large step forward into a lunge and then push back through the heel of the lunging leg to return to the start position.
- Reset yourself and lunge forward with the other leg. Brace your core throughout and keep the weight pressed firmly over your head.

⏱ **1:1**
(but controlled)

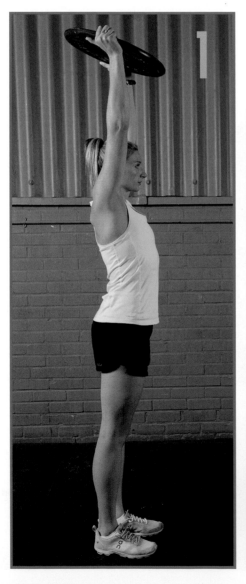

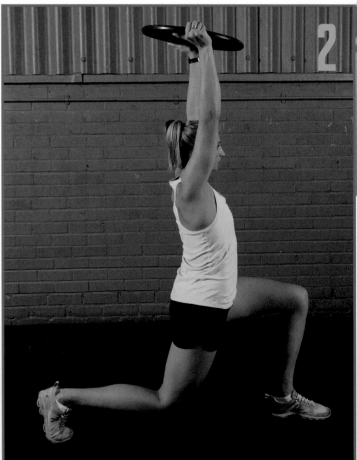

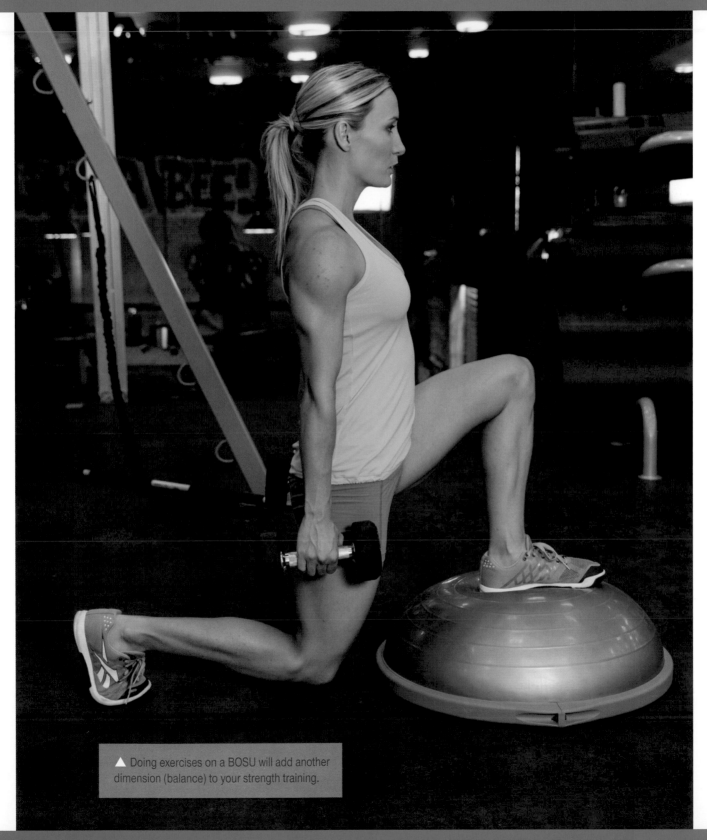

▲ Doing exercises on a BOSU will add another dimension (balance) to your strength training.

⏱ 1:1
(but controlled)

Plié squat with dumbbells

■ Stand with your feet wider than shoulder-width and turned out, making sure your feet and knees are similarly angled. Hold the dumbbells with your knuckles facing away from you beside your hips.

■ Bend your legs to plié and then extend them to stand back up.

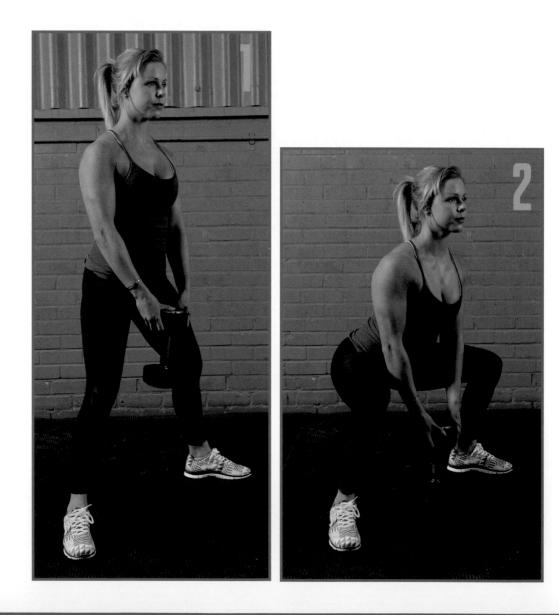

Dead lift

- Squat down with your feet under the bar and take hold of it, using an equally spaced knuckles-on-top grip. Maintain the natural curves of your spine and keep your head up.
- Straighten your legs to start to move the bar upward, keeping your arms long and the bar close to your shins (don't pull with your arms).
- Extend your hips to stand fully upright up with the bar across the front of your thighs.
- To return the bar to the floor, bend your legs and, keeping your head up, lower it under control, hinging your torso forwards as you do so.
- Reset and repeat.

The dead lift is perhaps the most important exercise of all for women wanting to shape a great lower body and develop lean muscle for fat burning.

 TIP

Practise with a light bar or even a broomstick before you go heavier. You can perform the exercise with dumbbells as a way of progressing to the barbell dead lift. This is primarily a glutes and hamstrings exercise – do not use your arms, and keep your core braced throughout. It's one of the best exercises you can do to shape a great lower body and, because of the large numbers of muscles involved, it's likely to boost your metabolic rate, not only as a result of performing the exercise, but also long term by increasing your lean muscle mass.

TARGET MUSCLES AND FUNCTIONAL BENEFITS

- Glutes
- Quadriceps
- Hamstrings
- Back

⏱ 1:1

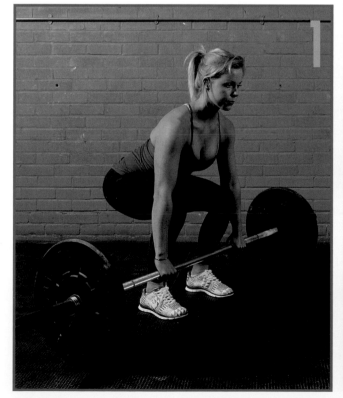

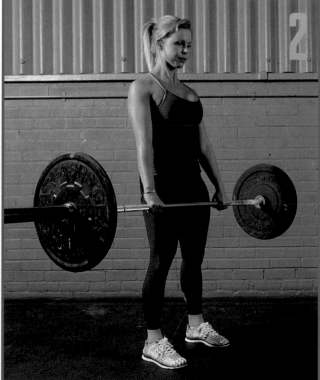

Squat

- Remove the bar from the squat racks, having set the racks at shoulder-height (you can also use a Smith machine – see page 162). Support it across the fleshy part of your rear shoulders (avoid contact with your top vertebrae).
- Pull the bar down onto your shoulders to fix it securely in place. Keep your head up and maintain the natural curves of your spine.
- Bend your knees to lower the weight. Keep your knees behind your toes as you lower and stand back up.

1:1

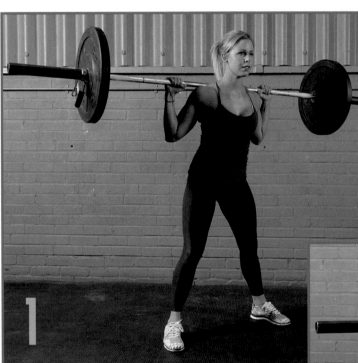

TIP

Push through the heels strongly on the way up and extend your hips as you near the top of the movement. Lower only as far as your flexibility (and strength) allows.

Your core must be braced throughout – see IAP (page 47).

As with the dead lift, the exercise can be learned with a broomstick and performed with dumbbells.

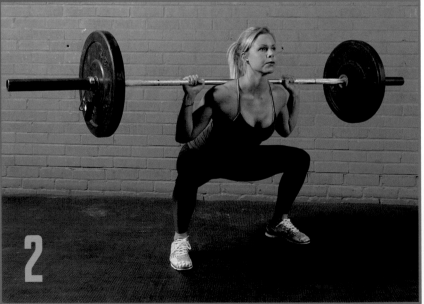

Seated shoulder press

- Sit on an exercise bench with your feet evenly spaced on the floor.
- Lift the dumbbells to shoulder-height (with your knuckles facing behind you).
- Maintaining the natural curves of your spine, press the weights to arms' length, bringing them close together at the top of the arc.
- Lower under control.

TARGET MUSCLES AND FUNCTIONAL BENEFITS

- Front of shoulders
- Triceps

 1:1

TIP

The exercise can also be performed one arm at a time (called the 'alternate' press).

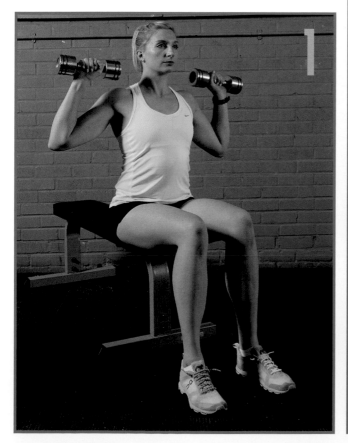

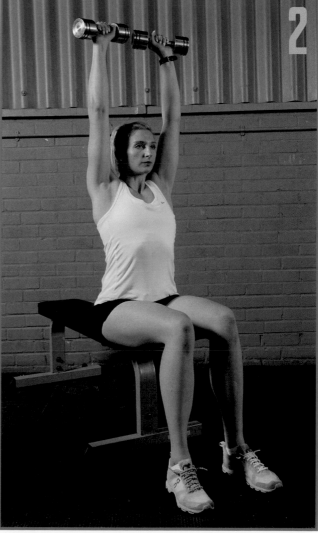

🏋 Ready, get set, go!

▶ Your resistance training plan starts here!

You'll now be familiar with all the exercises that you'll use for the first 12-week training programme. If you have any doubts, contact a personal trainer or other suitably qualified person. It could be worth spending a couple of sessions just going through the exercises with them and learning them, so that when you come to the programmes you'll be confident with what to do.

The first 6 weeks of this programme are divided into two 'prepare to resist' phases and are designed to ready you for future, more intense workouts. They are characterised by progressive body weight training. In week 7 – the start of the two 'resisting – intermediate' phases – there's an increase in intensity with the introduction of greater levels of resistance for you to train with, i.e. weight to lift. These phases will specifically develop your resistance training fitness and ready you for the more intense (in terms of weight lifted and resistance) workouts that follow in Chapter 5. Different training systems are introduced to further progress strength and fitness and increase lean muscle building and therefore fat burning potential – and to keep you from getting bored! They also introduce some of the weight training exercises that will be key to the subsequent 12-week programme in Chapter 5. It's all about building a base of confidence, strength and improved body awareness, control and functional movement.

▶ Chapter 4 Training Blocks

PREPARE TO RESIST
1 Weeks 1–3 Prepare to resist 1
2 Weeks 4–6 Prepare to resist 2

RESISTING – INTERMEDIATE
3 Weeks 7–9 Resisting – intermediate 1
4 Weeks 10–12 Resisting – intermediate 2

KEEP A RECORD OF YOUR TRAINING

Keeping a record of all your workouts will inform you so much about how your training is going and how well you are doing. This will also act as a great source of motivation when you look back on all those workouts that you have completed. Your diary entries (whether old-fashioned and in a paper diary or on a computer or app) should record the session and then the reps and weight of exercises (where relevant) that you complete. You should also record any comments you may have – for example, how you felt, whether you felt ready to move up a weight, whether an exercise was particularly difficult and so on. You could set up a social media page to motivate yourself and others through your achievements and your body transformation – more of which in Chapter 8.

NUMBER OF WORKOUTS PER WEEK – REST AND RECOVERY

Each of the weekly programmes requires you to perform 3–5 workouts a week. Resistance training requires rest and adaptive recovery. You might think that more sessions will get you more results, but what really counts is the quality of your training and the quality of your rest, recovery and nutrition. It's in the time when you are not training that your body responds to the stimulus of your workouts. If you don't allow enough time for recovery, you run the risk of compromised training adaptation and overtraining. Simply put, you won't burn as much fat or shape the body you desire and you could actually feel tired and not invigorated by your workouts.

Note: If you do feel more tired than normal and your muscles (and mind) have not fully recovered from the workouts prescribed, feel free to reduce the training loads – i.e. cut down on the numbers of reps and sets and even add an extra day's rest into the training programme. It's all about completing the programme and training for the bigger picture. Obviously don't keep missing sessions, though! If you do happen to do this (tut-tut!), forget the one you missed and do the next one in the sequence,

▶ Do you need a personal trainer?

I'd advise that you use the services of a personal trainer (or similar fitness/sports professional) if you are unsure about your fitness and the performance of any of the exercises and workouts in this book. Just make sure you find one who will really help you resistance train and who appreciates the benefits of kettlebells, barbells and body weight exercises for you. It's best to find a PT who practises what they preach – perhaps try to find a female PT who is fully converted and living proof of the benefits of resistance training. Most of the case study women featured in the book have used a PT at some time.

Emily Lingard

SIX-STONE WEIGHT LOSS

Emily Lingard had a triumph with weight training, culminating with an amazing 6-stone weight loss!

'People have always been shocked at my transformation. Those who didn't know me when I was at my heaviest of 14 stone 6lbs (92kg) wouldn't even recognise me now, but it hasn't been easy and identifying the cause of my weight gain was key to working out how to combat it and make the change.

'I can't blame it on my upbringing. I had a great childhood, I was always given home-cooked meals and no junk food was allowed in the house. The only thing we were allowed after dinner was fruit and we could choose one treat a week! My mum was really into fitness, never smoked, rarely drank and tried to instil the same attitude in my sister and me. While I wasn't sporty, I was massively into dancing – tap, ballet and jazz. But when I was 10 we moved and I had to stop dancing, as we couldn't find a dance school to the same standard. Luckily my metabolism was amazing and I stayed pretty slim for over a decade. At 21 I went to live in Spain, where I lived with a foodie and that's when I started eating everything! As my mum put it (and I'm not offended) I went away a swan and came back three years later a goose!

'When I graduated, I rented a flat near to my family home and, not having any local friends, joined a gym. I ramped up hours of cardio and exercise classes and joined Weight Watchers for a few months to keep occupied – losing around a stone in the process. I continued doing the same routine in the gym but nothing was changing and the weight remained. That was until a rather wonderful PT from the gym told me he could change all that with no cardio, clean eating and weights. Introduced to kettlebells, I became addicted, racking up hours a week swinging here, there and everywhere! I overhauled my diet to clean, healthy whole food and started dropping weight and changing my shape within a couple of months.

'I changed my entire routine to lifting weights five days a week. The results were pretty quick to follow and after losing 2 stone (13kg) in a year I decided I would take it a step further and compete, to enter fitness model shows. That's where even more change came. I quickly learnt about eating six times a day, splitting my workouts down to focus on building up certain areas and working to a macro split of proteins, carbohydrates and fats. I also discovered that having a coach with experience in competing would teach me more than anyone else would, not only about diet and training but also about the industry as a whole.

'But even if you don't want to compete and just want to feel good about yourself I can honestly say anyone can do it! I have a full-time job while fitting in morning cardio and evening training. The key is getting organised! I prepare my food at least two days in advance, box it all up into Tupperware and make sure I eat every three hours.

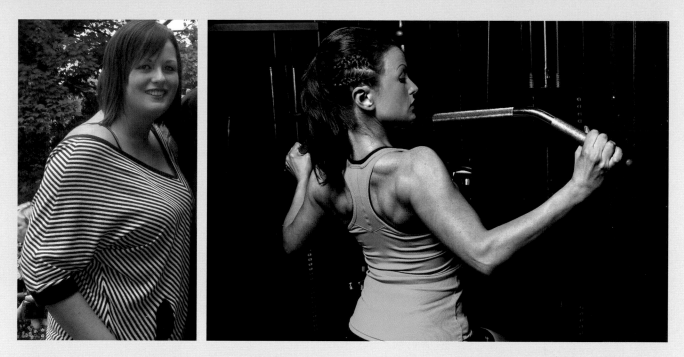

▲ Emily Lingard, before and after.

'My diet is broken down into six meals a day and is a combination of protein, carbohydrates and fats. In terms of carbs I eat varying quantities of oats, sweet potato, rice cakes and rice. On my rest day I reduce my carbs and load up on healthy fats instead, which means I get to eat avocados and nuts, which I love. My protein sources are lean meats, such as chicken, turkey, lean steak mince and white fish. I use various seasonings so it's not bland and add in lots of green vegetables. I also supplement with BCAAs and a range of vitamins [see Chapter 7 for more information] but I would recommend everyone use an intra-workout drink.

'I understand that my lifestyle isn't for everyone – I train and eat with a very specific goal in mind. So what about if you just want to look and feel good? My main advice would be give yourself time to see results – 6–12 weeks is ideal. Don't follow any fad diets, they may work in the short term, but making sensible food choices is better in the long term and will actually cost you less money and more importantly, add more value to your health. Keep a track of what you're eating and make sure it's predominantly protein then carbs and then fats.

'When it comes to training – lift weights, ladies! I understand it can be daunting and I've been in the position where I've been put off walking into a male dominated area of the gym but once you're there you will feel so empowered!

So good luck, go kick some booty and build yourself a body you're proud of!'

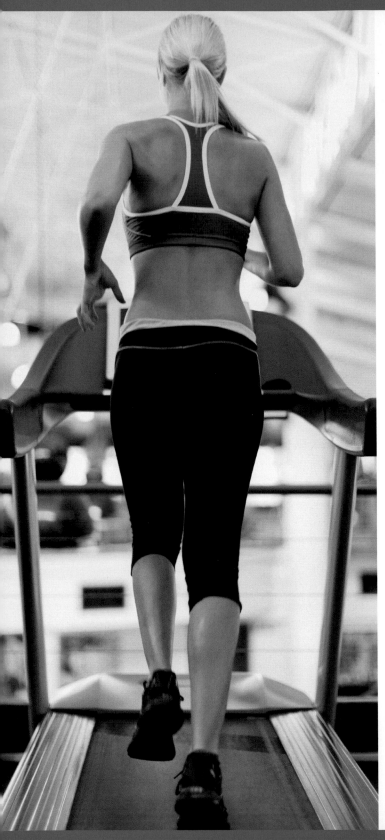

A note on CV training

Resistance training is important for calorie burning and building lean muscle and elevating metabolic rate. The calorie burning function is perhaps not something that many people attribute to resistanace training. Too much CV training, however, can actually work against these training goals. This is because it can result in a potential lowering of metabolic rate, due to reduction in muscle mass (your body 'eats' into its lean mass for energy and, with less lean muscle, your metabolic rate decreases).

Pedalling for hours and hours over numerous workouts on a stationary bike, although developing basic aerobic fitness, is in many ways taking other perhaps more important aspects of fitness nowhere. What do I mean? Well, exercise bike pedalling – although, of course, better than no exercise at all – will do little to combat osteoporosis, for example, because to get the exercise bone-bolstering benefits you have to support your body weight with or without resistance. Nor will stationary cycling build functional strength across your body, as it only targets your legs and then only certain parts. Indoor cycling is also lacking in mental stimulation and can be far from fun! I believe that resistance training is far more engaging of mind and muscle and can significantly contribute to weight loss and improve movement, balance and strength, with far more everyday benefits.

For those of you who need more convincing, resistance workouts can develop CV fitness and burn significant numbers of calories, particularly if recoveries are kept short and the bouts of exercise performed (intervals) are done at a medium to high intensity. Many of the workouts

◀ There is a place for steady-state CV training but for this book's purposes it is kept to a minimum.

you'll find in this book do just this. In fact they are typical of the Circuit Training or High Intensity Training (HIT) workouts that you may have heard about or even tried at your local gym. HIT has been around since fitness training began (i.e. as circuit training). Many of the workouts you'll be performing reflect the HIT/circuit way of training and with them comes a high calorific burn. You could potentially burn 500 calories during a 45-minute HIT workout.

The book includes complementary CV workouts in the training plans. These are specific CV workouts, provided as a variation from the resistance workouts that you'll follow, and they are there to provide you with some additional specific health and fitness benefits. Regardless of your starting point, the workouts are designed to add to your resistance training and not detract from it. Running is the preferred option, preferably outdoors. This activity is weight bearing, works virtually all the muscles in your body and is, of course, very easy to access.

The complementary CV workouts are often interval based. This type of workout can burn calories at a higher rate than steady-paced aerobic ones and will have a greater strengthening effect as you have to put more effort into your running stride, for example, to run faster. They will also create a greater after-burn. The CV workouts also include some sprint sessions. Sprinting is a high metabolic cost activity and works virtually every muscle in your body, burning fat and building a lean body fast.

None of these complementary CV workouts will take long to complete and because they involve running you'll be able to do them virtually anywhere and at any time.

You'll see from the workouts in the tables that follow that, where relevant, a designated Rate of Perceived Exertion (RPE) is given. Please study these guidelines to pace your effort. Note that as you get fitter you will be able

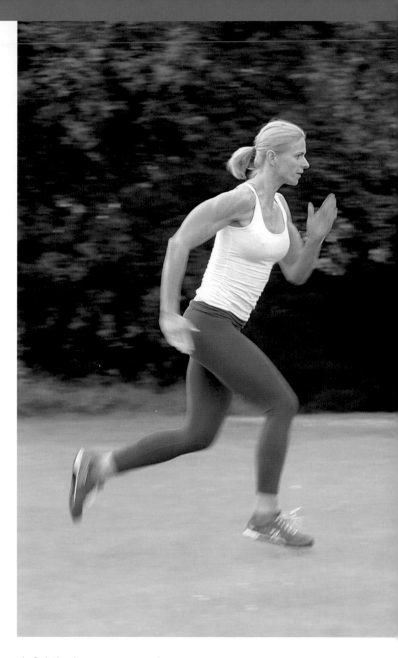

▲ Spinting is a great way to give your metabolism a high-powered boost.

to tolerate higher levels of exercise intensities, thus you should always be mindful of readjusting your RPE levels accordingly.

RATE OF PERCEIVED EXERTION – A WAY OF JUDGING AND CONTROLLING YOUR EXERCISE EFFORT

When I'm training a client, I'll often ask them to rate how they feel in terms of effort on a scale of 1–10, where 1 is 'easy, no effort at all' and 10 is 'flat out, ready to fall over'! Here's the RPE scale in more detail:

1   No effort at all.

2-4   Very easy, light aerobic exercise. Holding a conversation while exercising is no problem. Long period of effort possible.

5-7   More difficult exercise; breathing becomes heavier and you'll start sweating. Difficult to hold a conversation. More anaerobic than aerobic, but a relatively long period of effort is possible.

8-9   Very difficult to exercise; breathing is heavy and you will be sweating profusely. Totally anaerobic, only possible to sustain for a few minutes. You'll struggle to get the odd word out, if at all.

10   Flat out exercise. No chance of talking. Sweating very heavily, if part of a sprint at the end of a longer, slower effort. Also reached if an exercise is performed near to 100 per cent for 3–10 seconds, i.e. a sprint or heavy load set of squats, although you will recover quickly in this case.

Suggested RPEs are provided for the CV workouts in the workout programmes and for some of the circuit training based workouts. The latter will specifically target your anaerobic and aerobic energy systems and heart and lungs. Do try to maintain the rates indicated. If you do this, you should be able to complete each session. This will allow both constant progression and for your fitness to systematically and safely progress. You'll also gain satisfaction and confidence as you complete workout after workout.

WHY USE RPE?
You could use a heart rate monitor and work to designated heart rate ranges, for example, and although nowadays the kit required to do this is relatively inexpensive, you can control your workout effort very simply with RPE.

   The beauty of RPE is that a 'level 6' will always be a 'level 6', even if you are having a good (or bad) workout day. With heart rate training, an off day could see you struggle to keep within a targeted range.

⬛ Training systems

In Chapter 3, various different training systems were identified. You'll be using most of these in the training programmes in this chapter and the subsequent workout chapters. I have used abbreviations of their names for the workouts; here they are as a recap:

SS	Simple sets
SuS	Supersets*
DS	Drop sets
GS	Giant sets
P	Pyramids
	DS = descending pyramid,
	AS = ascending pyramid
SR	Split routine
NL	Negatives
FR	Forced reps
EDT	Escalating density training
GVT	German volume training
CT	Circuit training
CRT	Circuit resistance training
AMRAP	As many reps as possible
Weights	Weights (or predominantly weights based workout)

*Complex training (combining plyometric jumping type exercises and weights exercises into sets is included here).

▶ Warming up and cooling down

Before your workout, perform 5 minutes of CV exercise, such as jogging or skipping. Then perform functional movements for all body parts, such as marching on the spot, heel raises, lunges, arm swings and trunk rotations.

After your workout, you should perform some gentle CV work for 2–5 minutes and then lightly stretch all major muscles. I recommend that you do stretches to increase your range of movement separately from the resistance workouts specified in the book. This is because tired, post-workout muscles are not so easily stretched and can be more prone to strain. Any stretches performed in your cool down should therefore be relatively gentle. Focus on the main muscles in your torso, shoulders and legs and hold for 10–15 seconds each, but don't go for maximum range.

▶ Too easy or too hard?

Whether you find the workouts initially too easy or too hard will depend on your existing level of fitness and relevant exercise experience. I have deliberately started the programme with an assumption that you'll have a medium level of fitness. However, if you do initially find the workouts tough, reduce the number of reps or sets or increase the recovery so you can manage. The workouts should be 'comfortably manageable' initially.

▶ Workout types and names

The majority of workouts in this chapter are based on the HIT principle, being designed to be dynamic, stop-start, interval based workouts that target the majority of your body's larger muscles with compound movements. These HIT workouts, such as the 'All-body blast' and 'Lower body metabolic blaster', have names that aptly describe what they are designed to do. In Table 6 you'll find these and other named workouts and a brief description of their goals. These are used in this and the next chapter. For more detail on HIT training, see Chapter 6.

Workout names and brief description

TABLE 6

WORKOUT NAME	DESCRIPTION
Legs, bottom and core	A circuit focusing on these body parts – workouts get tougher across the first 6 weeks of the plan.
Lower body metabolic blaster	A circuit based workout that includes dynamic exercises, such as the Speed skater, Squat with rear kick and Jump squat. A workout designed to have a high metabolic (calorie burning) cost.
Lower body metabolic blaster – all angle attack	A variation on the previous workout – this one includes exercises that work your lower limbs in multiple directions and using different muscles. Exercises include the Plié squat and Side lunges. A very functional workout.
All-body workout blast	A circuit based workout that employs upper, lower and core exercises to get you into great shape.
Weights – learning technique	To ensure you progress safely when the levels of resistance increase, workouts are included that are all about learning how to perform the key moves in your next training phase. N.B. Don't be afraid to seek expert advice from a PT or other suitably qualified fitness professional should you need it.
Weights	These progressively and systematically use different training systems and different loads to maximise the development of your lean body mass and functional strength.
Body weight and weights session Stability emphasis	These workouts include full body exercises that work your body from top to bottom and bottom to top. The particular emphasis is on dumbbell exercises – for example, the Single leg biceps curl to Overhead press.
Fat burning power-up	These workouts purposely combine weights exercises with plyometric (jumping) exercises to make for a very dynamic and high metabolic cost workout.
Dynamic superset Barbell/dumbbell plyo combo) Chapter 5	These supersets (paired exercises) are designed to have a high metabolic cost and lean muscle building function. They combine weights exercises with jumping ones (the weights exercises using medium to heavy weights).
Barbell and suspension trainer superset Chapter 5	Similar to the above but a quick-fire repetition of suspension trainer and barbell exercises in one set.
BOSU™ blast Chapter 5	A simple set of exercises performed in quick succession on a BOSU™.
Kettlebell dominant all-body workout Chapter 5	Self-explanatory!

▶ A guide to what weight to lift

In the workout tables in this chapter you'll see that the exercises have been given a suggested load to work with, i.e. medium weight, heavy weight and so on. These follow the rep ranges suggested here. Note that these are guidelines only, to give you an idea as to the weight you should be lifting each workout. These require that the last reps in each set are difficult to complete but with good form. In reality, they will vary slightly between individuals because of previous weight training familiarity (exercises and exercise system, for example) and motivation.

A GUIDE TO WHAT WEIGHT TO LIFT

Weight to lift	Rep range	Approx % of 1RM
Light weight	10–20 plus	20–50%
Light/medium weight	8–12	50–60%
Medium weight	6–10	60–70%
Medium/heavy weight	4–8	70–80%
Heavy weight	3–6	80–90%
Heavy/very heavy weight	3–1	90–100%

TAKE A SELFIE

Take a selfie that shows off your physique – don't be shy now! Stick this somewhere prominent or in an accessible folder on your phone. Take another every week or every month should you wish, and definitely after the completion of this block of training. Why do I ask you to do this? Well, to see the changes that the workouts and the plan are having on your body.

Following certain pages and people on social media who are on the same journey as you or have successfully travelled it can be ideal motivation. Why not follow the women whose case studies are featured in this book? You could also set up your own social media pages so that you can inspire others and be motivated to keep up your training at the same time. After all, you won't want to let your followers down!

It's also important that you try to get your body composition measured (these tests are often available at your gym), specifically your lean vs fat mass and their distribution across your body. Over the course of the training programme, your fat weight should decline and your lean weight increase. Weighing yourself on the scales alone could give a false reading of your body's actual healthy weight and composition. This is because it's possible that you may gain the 'right' weight (lean muscle) as you go through the workouts.

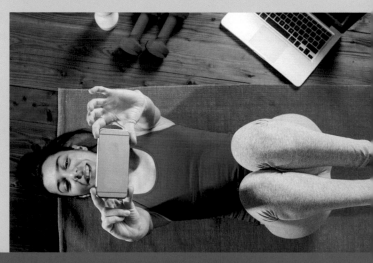

☎ Weeks 1–4 Prepare to resist 1

week 1

SESSION	TRAINING SYSTEM	EXERCISES AND RPE (Where relevant)	OTHER COMMENTS
1	CT SS 3 x 10 All-body workout	• Squat; Press-up; Ab crunch; Triceps dips; Glute bridge; Lunge (10 on each leg, i.e. 20 in each set) • Take 60sec at the end of each circuit • Work at a steady pace • RPE 5–7	• You kick off with a body weight workout that targets all your muscles.
2	CV Running	• 2 x 7min intervals at RPE 5–7 • Rest period – walk recovery 4min at RPE 1	• Stick to the designated effort levels. • Remember you're just getting started.
3	CT SS 3 x 10 Lower body metabolic blaster	• Squat into knee lift (alternate knee lift on each rep); Press-ups; Groiners; Speed skater; Squat with rear kick (alternating kick on each rep); Glute bridge • 20sec between exercises • Take 60sec at the end of each circuit • RPE 5–7 (may get nearer to 8, but don't push further; if you feel you are in the RPE 8 area, then give yourself more rest)	• This is a faster paced workout as the exercises are more dynamic and lend themselves to being performed at faster paces. The recovery is 20sec, but if this is too short, give yourself more recovery time so you can perform the sets in one go – rhythmically, correctly and fluently.
4	CT SS 3 x 12 Legs, bottom and core	• Side lunge (12 L&R); Plié squat (no weight); Scissors; Plank with leg lift (5 on right and 5 on left each set); Russian twist; Squat • 20sec between exercises and sets • Take 45sec at the end of each circuit • RPE 5–7	• More different exercises – you'll soon get used to all the movements required.

Your first week's training is all about getting used to working out and being able to handle your own body weight. The mix of body weight exercises will work all your major muscles and boost your metabolism. Try not to perform circuits on consecutive days. You could take a day off after session 3, if you followed the workouts over a 5-day period in the order provided.

2

SESSION	TRAINING SYSTEM	EXERCISES AND RPE (Where relevant)	OTHER COMMENTS
1	CT SS 4 x 10 All-body workout	• Squat; Press-up: Ab crunch; Triceps dips; Glute bridge; Lunge (10 on each leg, i.e. 20 in each set) • 30sec between exercises • Take 60sec at the end of each set • RPE 5–7	• This is an escalation on the similar circuit performed in Week 1. Keep to the RPE.
2	CV Running	• 3 x 5min intervals at RPE 5–7 • Rest periods – 3min walk recovery at RPE 1	• An extra 5min work period this week.
3	CT SS 3 x 12 Lower body metabolic blaster	• Squat into knee lift (alternate knee lift on each rep); Press-ups; Groiners; Speed skater; Squat with rear kick (alternate kick on each rep); Glute bridge • 20sec between exercises; go from one to the next • Take 60sec at the end of each circuit • RPE 5–7 (may get nearer to 8, but don't push further; if you feel you are in the RPE 8 area, give yourself more rest)	• A slight increase on last week's session.
4	CT SS 4 x 14 Legs, bottom and core	• Side lunge (14 L&R); Plié squat (no weight); Scissors; Plank with leg lift (7 on right and 7 on left each set), Russian twist; Squat: • 30sec between exercises • Take 45sec at the end of each circuit • RPE 5–7	• A bigger jump for this workout – an extra circuit of 14 reps. The rest period has been increased to help you get through it!

Your second week's training is more or less a repeat of week 1, albeit with increased intensity and volume. You need to get familiar with the exercises and get into a rhythm. The aim at this stage is to develop a body used to all-body exercises and to develop good local muscular endurance and strength. The intensity of the workouts is designed to turn up your body's metabolic processes so that you become a better calorie burner.

3

SESSION	TRAINING SYSTEM	EXERCISES AND RPE (Where relevant)	OTHER COMMENTS
1	CT SS 4 x 12 All-body workout	• Squat; Press-up: Ab crunch; Triceps dips; Glute bridge; Lunge (12 on each leg) • 20sec between exercises • Take 45sec at the end of each circuit • RPE 5–7/8	• Keep to a steady pace but do push that bit harder than last week, so that you work out consistently at the top end of the designated RPE. • A shorter recovery and extra reps build on last week.
2	CV Running	• 4 x 90sec intervals at RPE 5–7/8 • Rest periods: Jog recovery 2min at RPE 2–4	• This is a tougher CV session than you've done so far – you need to commit to the intervals and allow yourself to go into the higher end of the RPE scale. Just hold enough back so you can complete the workout.
3	CT SS 4 x 10 Lower body metabolic blaster	• Squat into knee lift (alternate knee lift on each rep); Press-ups; Groiners; Speed skater; Squat with rear kick (alternate kick on each rep); Glute bridge, Squat jump • 20sec between exercises; go from one to the next and take 60sec at the end of each circuit. • RPE 5–7/8	• Note the addition of the squat jump. This exercise will up the intensity of the workout and elevate its metabolic cost. Allow yourself to go into RPE 8 territory. If it becomes too tough, increase your recovery.
4	CT SS 4 x 16 Legs, bottom and core	• Side lunge; Plié squat (no weight); Scissors; Plank with leg lift (8 on right and 8 on left, each set); Russian twist; Lunge walk; • For the lunge walk, perform 16 lunges continuously forwards if space permits • 20sec between exercises • Take 45sec at the end of each circuit • RPE 5–7/8	• Adding the walking lunges will add to the workout's intensity and help build greater leg strength.

Your third week's training adds more exercises to the circuits and provides probably your toughest CV challenge so far. The intensity factor is well and truly turned up. Again, try to stick to the suggested RPEs, get through the sessions and complete all that is required.

SESSION	TRAINING SYSTEM	EXERCISES AND RPE (Where relevant)	OTHER COMMENTS
1	CT SS 5 x 10 All-body workout	• Squat; Press-up: Ab crunch; Triceps dips; Glute bridge; Lunge (10 on each leg, i.e. 20 in each set); • 30sec between exercises and sets • Take 45sec at the end of each circuit • RPE 5–7	• Another circuit adds to the workout's volume. By now, your body should be responding well to the training.
2	CV Running	• 8 x 60sec efforts • Intervals at RPE 5–7/8 • Rest periods 90sec at RPE 2–4/5 • Jog recovery	• This is a tough CV workout. As last week, you need to commit to the intervals and allow yourself to go into the higher end of the RPE scale. The recoveries will also be tougher as you will have less time to recover from each effort. If you need to, take longer, but aim to complete the workout at the speed required to sustain the effort RPE.
3	CT SS 4 x 12 Lower body metabolic blaster	• Squat into knee lift (alternate knee lift on each rep); Press-ups; Groiners; Speed skater; Squat with rear kick (alternate kick on each rep); Glute bridge; Squat jump • 10sec between exercises • Take 45sec at the end of the circuit • RPE 5–7/8	• Another 2 reps to each exercise ups the intensity that bit more.
4	CT SS 4 x 18 Legs, bottom and core	• Side lunge; Plié squat (no weight); Scissors; Plank with leg lift (9 on right and 9 on left, each set), Russian twist, Lunge walk • 20sec between exercises • Take 60sec at the end of each circuit • RPE 5–7/8	• This workout is a repeat of last week's – your training needs to be progressive and not jump too quickly to higher levels.

This is the final week of phase 1 of your training in the 'prepare to resist' section and the intensity and volume has increased significantly from the first week. In the next 4-week phase, exercise selection changes gradually and some are performed with added resistance. This is all in preparation for the heavier load exercises that follow later.

Weeks 5-6 Prepare to resist 2

This phase introduces added resistance to many of the exercises you performed in the first 'prepare to resist' phase. This will start to really build that increased lean body mass that will burn calories 24/7. As usual, the emphasis is on compound exercises that recruit lots of your body's muscles – exercises that have a high metabolic cost. The CV sessions continue to build.

week 5

SESSION	TRAINING SYSTEM	EXERCISES AND RPE (Where relevant)	OTHER COMMENTS
1	CT SS 6x 10 Legs, bottom and core – all angle attack!	• Plié squat; Scissors; Side lunges (10 in each direction); Single leg squat (10 on each leg); Russian twist; Squat with front kick (alternate kick on each rep) • 30sec between exercises and sets • Take 90sec at the end of each circuit • RPE 5–7	• The exercises in this workout will challenge your mind and muscles as you move sideways and dynamically and with strength and power.
2	CV Running	• 9 x 30sec effort intervals at RPE 5–7/8 • Rest periods: 40sec • Jog recovery at RPE 2–4/5	• This is a tough CV workout; as with the similar previous ones, you will need to commit to the intervals and allow yourself to go into the higher end of the RPE scale. The recoveries will also be tougher as you have less time. If running on the roads or using a running track, try to match the distances you achieve on each rep.
3	CT SS 4 x 12 Lower body metabolic blaster	• Squat into knee lift (alternate knee lift on each rep); Brazilian crunch; Squat with rear kick (alternate kick on each rep); Glute bridge, Squat jump; In and out • 10sec between exercises • Take 60sec at the end of each circuit • RPE 5–7/8	• This is another dynamic workout that will get your metabolism revved up.
4	SuS 4 x 30sec/ exercise Legs, bottom and core	• SuS 1: Reverse crunch and Plank with leg lift (keep alternating legs lifted) • SuS 2: Squat and Glute bridge • SuS 3: Press-up and Triceps dip • SuS 4: Squat with rear kick and Squat with front kick (alternate kicks and lift on each rep) • 4 x 30sec on each exercise in each SuS, no rest between the exercises • 20sec between each superset • RPE 5–7/8	• This is another high-intensity workout.

The intensity pushes up higher this week as we move towards the next phase of training.
By now, your muscles and metabolism will be responding well to the challenge of the workouts.

week 6

SESSION	TRAINING SYSTEM	EXERCISES AND RPE (Where relevant)	OTHER COMMENTS
1	CT SS 6 x 10 Legs, bottom and core plus all angle attack and Isometric exercises	• Plié squat; Scissors; Side lunges (10 in each direction); Single leg squat (10 on each leg); Russian twist; Squat with front kick (alternate kick on each rep) • 20sec between exercises and sets • RPE 5–7 • 3–5min recovery • Press-up plank and Wall squat 3 x 20sec holds • 30sec recovery between exercises	• The reduced recovery at the end of each set ups the intensity
2	CV Running	• 10 x 30sec intervals at RPE 5–7/8 • Rest periods 60sec at RPE 2–4/5 • Jog recovery	• An extra interval is added from last week's workout.
3	CT SS 4 x 12 Lower body metabolic blaster	• Squat into knee lift (alternate knee lift on each rep); Brazilian crunch; Squat with rear kick lift (alternate kick on each rep); Glute bridge, Squat jump; In and out • 10sec between exercises; go from one to the next and take 45sec at the end of each circuit • RPE 5–7/8	• A shorter recovery at the end of each circuit ups the intensity above the same workout performed last week.
4	SuS 4 x 30sec on each exercise Legs, bottom and core	• SuS 1: Reverse crunch and Plank with leg lift (keep alternating leg lifted) • SuS 2: Squat and Glute bridge • SuS 3: Press-up and Triceps dip • SuS 4: Squat with rear kick and Squat with front kick • RPE 5–7/8	• Perform in the same way as session 4 from last week's session.

Weeks 7-12 Intermediate 1 and 2

The workouts that follow are designed to exploit lean muscle. You'll switch over the course of the phases from circuit style training to predominately weight training, using progressively heavy weights on selected key exercises during workouts. Combo weight exercises are also introduced, which combine two or more exercises into one – for example, the all-body single leg curl to press, which targets virtually every muscle in your body. Swiss ball exercises are also introduced.

▶ Resisting Intermediate 1

week

SESSION	TRAINING SYSTEM	EXERCISES AND RPE (Where relevant)	OTHER COMMENTS
1	EDT All-body workout blast	• 3 x 5min blocks • Squats; Triceps dips; Russian twist • 40sec between blocks	• With EDT, it's all about maximum numbers of reps. Pace yourself in each block and record your scores to beat next time you repeat the workout.
2	Weights: Learning technique Swiss ball exercises	• Weights exercises: (barbell unless indicated otherwise) Squat; Seated shoulder press (dumbbells); Dead lift; Lunges (dumbbells only); Plié squat (dumbbells); Rear foot elevated split squat (dumbbells) • Start with just a light bar/dumbbells • 5min recovery • Swiss ball hamstring curl • 4 x 12 reps; 30sec between sets	• From now on, we start to introduce some of the weight training exercises that will be a key feature of this training programme. Many more are introduced in Chapter 5.
3	Weights: Learning technique	• Repeat workout 2. Don't try to lift too much yet – just focus on exercise technique.	
4	SS Weights session and body weight exercises	• Weights exercises: (barbell unless indicated otherwise) Squat; Seated shoulder press (dumbbells); Dead lift; Rear foot elevated split squat (dumbbells) • 3 x 8–10 light to medium weight • Body weight: Press-ups; Glute bridge: 3 x 10; Plank 3 x 20sec holds • Take a full recovery between exercises (resistance and body weight)	• You can start to slightly increase the weight you lift, but only if you are confident in your technique.
5	CV Running	• 2 x 8min intervals at RPE 5–7 • 4min jog recovery at RPE 2–4	• An easier session to make for a less intense overall week's workouts.

The resistance emphasis starts to change now, with the addition of key weights exercises and new training systems, such as EDT.

There are two weights workouts called 'Learning technique'. If you are familiar with the exercises, replace one of these with the specified weights session (workout 4). Keep one in for familiarity and to ease you into this new phase. Regardless of your training background, don't rush into lifting heavy weights – you need to build gradually (and master the techniques of each, where appropriate). At this stage, it's best to underestimate what you think you can lift as you need to get your body prepared for the more intense workouts that follow.

For those new to weight training, each session will need to be carefully progressed; just holding light dumbbells when performing the Rear foot elevated split squat, for example, will work your shoulders, upper arms and core, as well as working the exercise's main target muscles in your legs.
The benefits will be huge but you need to take small steps initially.

Give yourself a day between performing each of the weights based workouts (both learning and actual weights ones). There's also an extra workout this week to maintain the metabolic boosting accumulation of the training programme, although the total intensity of the week should be easier than previous ones.

SESSION	TRAINING SYSTEM	EXERCISES AND RPE (Where relevant)	OTHER COMMENTS
1	EDT **All-body workout blast**	• 3 x 5min blocks • Squats; Triceps dips; Russian twist • 40sec between blocks	• See if you can beat your scores from last week.
2	SS **Weights session and body weight exercises**	• Weights exercises (barbell unless otherwise indicated): Lunge; Seated shoulder press (dumbbells); Dead lift; Plié squat (dumbbell) • 3 x 8–10 light to medium weight medium • 5min recovery • Body weight: Press-ups; Glute bridge: 3 x 10; Toe taps 3 x 20; Press-up plank 3 x 20sec holds • Take 20sec between exercises	• A different combination of exercises from your last weights session.
3	CV **Running**	• 3 x 5min intervals at RPE 5–7 • 3min jog recovery at RPE 2–4	• Another option to keep your mind and muscles fresh and fitness gains coming.

SESSION	TRAINING SYSTEM	EXERCISES AND RPE (Where relevant)	OTHER COMMENTS
4	P **Weights session** SS **Body weight exercises**	• Weights exercises: (barbell unless otherwise indicated) Squat; Seated shoulder press (dumbbells); Dead lift; Rear foot elevated split squat (dumbbells) start with a very light weight and increase the resistance to a medium weight over the sets of your first pyramid workout • 5 minute recovery • Body weight: Scissors 3 x 20; Glute bridge 3 x 10; In and Out 3 x 20. Take 20sec recovery between exercises	• Your first pyramid session. Make sure you record the weights you lift.

You can now start to up the weights you lift, albeit gradually – hence the inclusion of the pyramid workout. Ensure that the last reps of each set are difficult but not impossible to perform, while maintaining good technique. The exercises are the same across the weights workouts to allow you to become consistent with their technique and so that you can begin to get a true feel of your lifting capabilities. The CV session – as with the week before – is designed to aid recovery and should therefore be performed at the specified RPE.

week

9

SESSION	TRAINING SYSTEM	EXERCISES AND RPE (Where relevant)	OTHER COMMENTS
1	SS **Lower body metabolic blaster**	• Squat into knee lift (alternate knee lift on each rep); Brazilian crunch; Squat with rear kick (alternate knee lift on each kick); Glute bridge; Squat jump; In and out • 4 x 30sec on each exercise and 30 sec recovery between each • Take 60sec at the end of each circuit • RPE 5–7/8 • 5min recovery • Feet elevated crunch; Scissors 3 x 20 • 30sec on 30sec off	• This session requires you to perform more reps than previous similar ones as you work for 30sec and not for a set number of reps. Control your effort. The length of recovery should be long enough to allow for a full-on commitment to each exercise.

Strength, coordination, balance, power and core strength all get specifically resistance trained this week, in a way that will be new to many of you. It's the aim of the programme to cover all muscular actions to make for truly functional fitness. Functional exercise that will make you fit and fab for life!

SESSION	TRAINING SYSTEM	EXERCISES AND RPE (Where relevant)	OTHER COMMENTS
2	SS Weights session	• Weights exercises (barbell unless otherwise indicated); Squat; Seated shoulder press (dumbbells); Dead lift; Lunges • 3 x 7–8 medium weight (this should be around 70% of your estimated 1RM) • Full recovery between exercises (resistance and body weight) • 5min recovery • Body weight: Brazilian crunch; Swiss ball hamstring curl: 3 x 10 • Take 30sec between exercises	• It's now time to really really start to lift a heavier weight in the medium range of strength types – so, as indicated, around 70% 1RM. The last few reps of the exercises may prove difficult to complete. If you feel you are going to 'fail' on a set, then take a longer recovery, or even split the set – i.e. stop, put the weight down, recover and restart to get each set completed. The number of weights exercises has been cut down to give you the best chance of completing the exercise with good strength levels.
3	CV Running	• 2 x 8min intervals at RPE 5–7 • 4min jog recovery at RPE 2–4	This is a recovery session between the weights workouts so you should keep within the RPEs noted.
4	SS Weights session and SS Body weight exercises	• Weights exercises (barbell unless otherwise indicated): Squat; Seated shoulder press (dumbbells); Dead lift; Rear foot elevated split squat (dumbbells) • 3 x 8–10 medium weight • Allow a full recovery between exercises • 5min recovery • Body weight: Press-ups; Glute bridge: 3 x 10 Press-up plank 3 x 20sec holds • Take 20sec between exercises	
5	SS Body weight and weights session Stability emphasis	• Weights exercises (all dumbbell): Single leg biceps curl to press; Rear foot elevated squat; Rear lunge with triceps extension; Plié squat; • 3 x 16 light weight (with the first three exercises, perform 8 reps off one leg and then 8 off other) • Take 45sec between exercises • 5min recovery • Body weight: Reverse curl to toe touch; Glute bridge; Plank • 3 x 20 first two exercises and 3 x 30sec holds for third • Take 30sec between exercises	New weights exercises are introduced. These tend to suit lighter weights, hence the higher number of reps compared to some previous weights workouts. There are body weight exercises too, to make for a substantial workout.

Resisting Intermediate 2

In this next phase, the principles of the last three weeks are continued, but there is a further increase in resistance in order to get you fully prepared for the workouts in Chapter 5.

week 10			
SESSION	**TRAINING SYSTEM**	**EXERCISES AND RPE** (Where relevant)	**OTHER COMMENTS**
1	**SS** **Lower body metabolic blaster**	• Squat into knee lift; Brazilian crunch; Squat with rear kick (alternate kick with each rep); Glute bridge; Squat jump; Burpee • 5 x 30sec on each exercise and 30sec recovery • RPE 7–9	• The introduction of the Burpee will really up the difficulty of this workout as it is a very high metabolic cost exercise. If the workout becomes too demanding, take more recovery and/or reduce the difficulty of the Burpee by omitting the jump and/or press-up.
2	**SuS Weights and body weight session**	• Weights exercises: • SuS 1: Dead lift and Squat; 4 x 8 x medium/heavy weight • SuS 2: Seated shoulder press (dumbbells) and Lunge with triceps extension; 4 x 12 with light to medium weight • SuS 3: Swiss ball hamstring curl and Wall sit 4 x 20 reps and 20sec hold • SuS 4: Lateral lunge and Jump squat • Move straight from one exercise to the next in each superset then take 60sec between each superset • 5min recovery • Plank 4 x 40sec hold with 20sec between reps	This workout covers all muscle actions and – where relevant – requires lifting the heaviest weights you have attempted so far.
3	**CV** **Running**	• 10 x 10sec sprints intervals at RPE 5–7/8 • 2min walk recovery at RPE 2–4 • This workout is quality-based and as such you should be fully recovered between sprints. This allows for a full-on commitment. Sprinting will target all your body's muscles and is a great way to burn calories and develop lean muscle. Warm up thoroughly before this session.	• A further note on sprinting: if you have not sprinted for a long time, it's recommended that you build up your speed on this and other sessions or through practice at other times. You could also perform a similar session on an exercise bike. If following this option, cycle for 20 seconds against a high resistance at over 110RPM and then pedal easy for 90sec at 70–80RPM at a low resistance for recovery. Do 12 reps.

SESSION	TRAINING SYSTEM	EXERCISES AND RPE (Where relevant)	OTHER COMMENTS
4	**P** **Weights session**	• Weights exercises (all barbell): Seated shoulder press (dumbbells); Dead lift; Lunges • 10 x light weight • 8 x medium weight • 6 x medium/heavy weight • 4 x heavy weight • 5min recovery • Body weight: Russian twist 4 x 20; Press-up plank 3 x 20sec holds; Scissors: 4 x 30 • Take a full recovery between all exercises	• You may need a training partner on hand for this workout as it's time to use heavier weights over this ascending pyramid. A partner can assist you and also spot for you, i.e. help you lift the dumbbells/bar/support you if you encounter difficulties. If you don't have this option available, don't do the 4 x heavy reps and go for a second set of 6 at the medium/heavy weight. You could also use a Smith machine – where relevant, see Chapter 5.
5	**SS** **Body weight exercises** **SS** **Weights and body weight session** **Stability emphasis**	• Weights exercises: • Single leg biceps curl to press; Rear foot elevated squat; Rear lunge with triceps extension; Plié squat; Lunge with weight held over head; • 4 x 16 light weight (with the first three exercises, perform 8 reps from one leg and then 8 from other) • Take 45sec between exercises • 5min recovery • Body weight; Reverse curl to toe touch; Glute bridge; Press-up plank • 3 x 20 first two exercises and 3 x 30sec holds for the third • Take 30sec between exercises	• The extra circuit will add to the workout's difficulty over last week's.

A further progression in resistance this week with new exercises and some heavier lifting.

SESSION	TRAINING SYSTEM	EXERCISES AND RPE (Where relevant)	OTHER COMMENTS
1	**SuS Fat burning power-up**	• SuS 1: Barbell squat 3 x 8 medium weight and Jump squat x 8 • SuS 2: Barbell lunge 3 x 8 lunge (medium weight 6 off left and right leg) and Lunge jump 3 x 12 • SuS 3: Triceps dips and Press-ups 3 x 12 • SuS 4: Plank with leg lift (8 on right and 8 on left) and Crunch 3 x 16 • Full recovery between exercises, but remember that with supersets you move straight from the first to the second exercise	• The first of two supersets to use a specific combination of weights and plyometric (jumping) exercises in the programme. • These workouts are very good at targeting the fast twitch muscle fibres that stimulate lean muscle development.
2	**SuS Weights, dynamic weights and body weight exercises**	• Weights exercises: (barbell unless otherwise indicated) • SuS 1: Dead lift and Squat; 4 x 6 x medium/heavy weight • SuS 2: Seated shoulder press (dumbbells) and Lunge with triceps extension (dumbbells); 4 x 12 with light to medium weight • SuS 3: Rear foot elevated split squat and Lateral lunge (dumbbell); 4 x 12 light to medium weight • SuS 4: Swiss ball hamstring curl and Wall sit; 4 x 20 reps and 20sec hold	• A further superset training option.
3	**CV**	• Easy 20min run at RPE 2–4	• This is a recovery session so stick to the RPE.
4	**P Weights session**	• Weights exercises (all barbell): Squat; Seated shoulder press (dumbbells); Dead lift • 10 x light weight • 8 x medium weight • 6 x medium/heavy weight • 2 x 4 x heavy weight • 5min recovery • Body weight: Russian twist 4 x 20; Press-up plank 3 x 30sec holds; Scissors: 4 x 30 • Take 20sec between exercises	• As with the similar previous sessions, if you don't have a training partner to assist then don't do the 2 x 4 x heavy reps and go for a second set of 6 at the medium/heavy weight. • As before, you could use a Smith machine.

week 11

SESSION	TRAINING SYSTEM	EXERCISES AND RPE (Where relevant)	OTHER COMMENTS
5	**SS** **Body weight and weights session** **Stability emphasis**	• Weights exercises (all dumbbell): Single leg biceps curl to press; Rear foot elevated squat; Rear lunge with triceps extension; Plié squat; Lunge with weight held over head • 3 x 12 light/medium weight (with the first three exercises, perform 6 reps off of one leg and 6 from the other) • 5min recovery • Body weight: Reverse curl to toe touch; Plank with alternate leg lift • 3 x 30sec with 30sec between exercises	• The reps and number of exercises have dropped from last week's session but the idea is that you increase the weight you lift on the exercises where relevant, to increase the strength component of the workout.

By now you should really be seeing and feeling the benefits of a resistance trained body – you'll be functionally fit, leaner and stronger and your body's calorie burning furnace will be turned up high!

SESSION	TRAINING SYSTEM	EXERCISES AND RPE (Where relevant)	OTHER COMMENTS
1	SuS Fat burning power-up	• Weights exercises: (barbell unless otherwise indicated) • SuS 1: Squat (medium/heavy weight x 8) and Jump squat 3 x 8 • SuS 2: Dumbbell lunge (medium/heavy weight 3 x 8) and Lunge jump 3 x 12; • 5min recovery • Body weight: • SuS 3: Triceps dip and Press-up 3 x 12 • SuS 4: Plank with leg lift and Crunch 3 x 16 (for plank, alternate left/right leg lifts) • Take 30sec between supersets	• An increase in the weights this week. For the first two supersets, there is a commensurate reduction in reps. Have a training partner on hand or use a Smith machine where relevant. Remember to move straight from one exercise to the next in each superset and then take your recovery.
2	SuS Weights session Dynamic weights and Body weight exercises	• Weights exercises: • SuS 1: Dead lift (barbell) and Squat (barbell) 4 x 8 x medium/heavy weight • SuS 2: Seated shoulder press (dumbbells) and Lunge with triceps extension (dumbbells); 4 x 12 with light to medium weight • SuS 3: Rear foot elevated split squat (dumbbells) and Lateral lunge (dumbbells); 4 x 8 medium weight • SuS 4: Swiss ball hamstring curl and Wall squat 4 x 20 reps and 20sec hold • Take 60sec between supersets	• Increase the weight lifted if you can.
3	CV Running	• Easy 20min run at RPE 2–4	• This is a recovery session so stick to the RPE.
4	SS Body weight and weights session Stability emphasis	• Weights exercises: (all dumbbell): Single leg biceps curl to press; Rear foot elevated squat; Rear lunge with triceps extension; Plié squat; Lunge with weight held over head • 3 x 16 light/medium weight (with the first three exercises, perform 8 reps off one leg and then 8 from other) • 5min recovery • Body weight: Scissors 3 x 20; Plank 3 x 30sec holds. Take 30sec between exercises	• Again, increase the weight lifted, where relevant, if you feel ready.

SESSION	TRAINING SYSTEM	EXERCISES AND RPE (Where relevant)	OTHER COMMENTS
5	CV Running	• 10 x 10sec sprints at RPE 7–9 • 2min walk recovery at RPE 2–4	• As before, with this session you could perform a similar workout on an exercise bike – if following this option, cycle for 20 seconds against a high resistance at over 110RPM and then pedal easy for 90sec at 70-80RPM at a low resistance as recovery. Do 15 reps.

Two CV sessions are included this week to make a change from the resistance emphasis, but note that sprinting is in fact a great resistance based workout option in its own right. On each and every stride you'll be overcoming 2–3 times and more of your body weight and targeting your fast twitch muscle fibres. These are the fibres that will increase your leanness and 24/7 fat burning capability (as well as strength and speed).

You're now ready for the next 12-week phase in Chapter 5. This programme really gets you to where resistance training will have its greatest effects on your body and metabolism. New exercises and new training systems are introduced and the emphasis shifts to lifting heavier weights.

5 PATH TO RESISTANCE 2

Training programme: Weeks 13 - 24

By now you're well and truly on your way to building a functionally strong fat-burning body. Now it's time to move up an extra gear with the next 12 weeks of the training programme, to completely benefit from what resistance training can offer.

In the workouts in this chapter you'll get to grips with a further full array of resistance training options. These include dynamic barbell exercises such as the Clean, suspension trainer exercises such as the Atomic press-up, and an array of kettlebell and BOSU™ exercises. All these will take your training to the next level and keep the development of that lean, fat-burning body turned up high. And because there are so many more new ways to train, your motivation will be kept high.

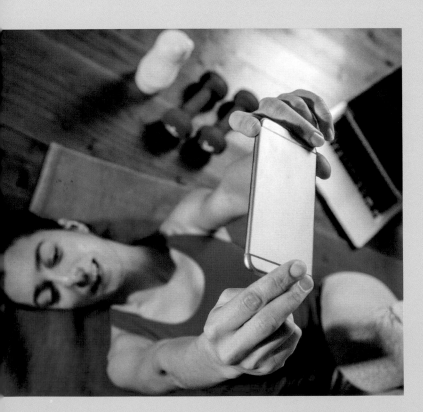

TAKE ANOTHER SELFIE

Just as you did at the start of the plan and then, at the very least, after the first 12 weeks of the training programme, take further selfies of the developing new you and stick these somewhere prominent to show just how far you have come. As before, you can take these weekly if you wish and upload them to your social media pages. And, as before, you can post comments as to how you are doing. Your followers will be growing! And remember to encourage other women to train with weights and other resistance training options.

Do try to get your body composition measured. By now, your fat weight should have declined and your lean mass increased. It's actually possible that you may have gained weight, although your fat mass has decreased, as muscle weighs more than fat; however, your body will be in much better shape and you'll be more toned.

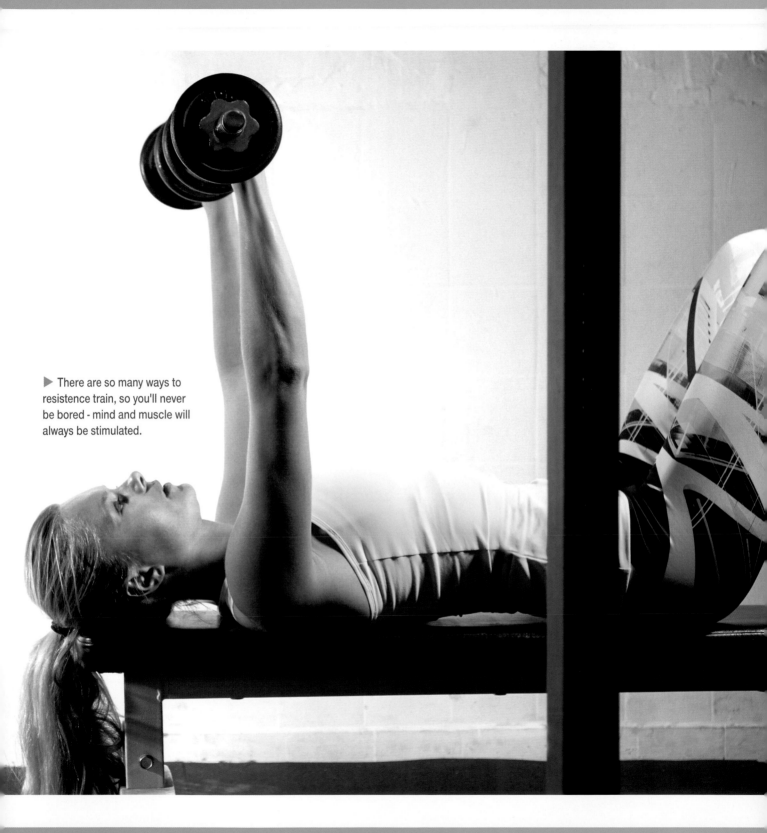

► There are so many ways to resistence train, so you'll never be bored - mind and muscle will always be stimulated.

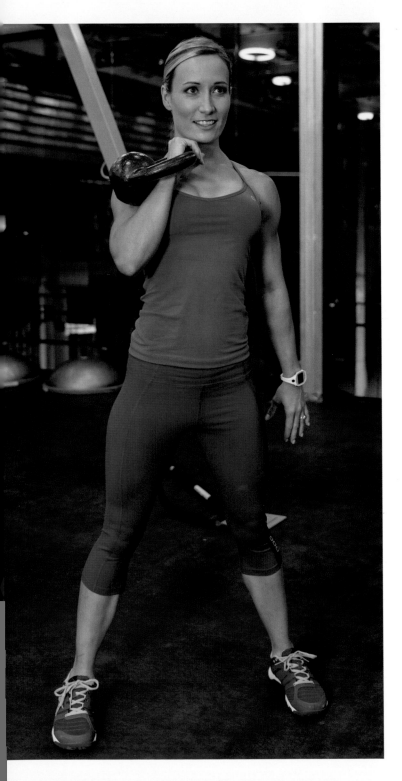

Training systems used for weeks 13–24

You'll now be familiar with many of the training systems after the first 12-week block, and you'll get to know more in this chapter! For a recap, see page 41-44.

NEW EXERCISES

You'll find the many new exercises used in this programme over the following pages of this chapter (many of those in the first 12-week block are also used). As before, they've been divided up where practical into lower, core and upper body and all-body exercises. The main difference is that the majority use added resistance – dumbbells, kettlebells and barbells. Many are very dynamic, such as the Barbell clean and Kettlebell swing. Again, a note is made of the muscles the exercises specifically target and, on occasions, the specific muscular action/s they use (i.e. isometric, plyometric etc) and their functional benefits. Exercise variations are also provided.

training equipment

Kettlebells

Kettlebells are a great way to resistance train and you'll find a number of exercises in this chapter. Originating from the former USSR, these 'cannonballs with handles' were made from old steam engines! Now you can use them to shape a great body with a range of dynamic moves. Because the mass of the kettlebell (the bell) moves below and around its handle, the demands placed on your entire body (even when performing an upper body exercise) are much greater than when performing a similar exercise with a dumbbell. Kettlebells can be carried, pressed, pushed, lifted and swung. Many have a high metabolic cost and will contribute significantly to developing a functional, low fat body by burning calories and shaping muscle.

LOWER BODY EXERCISES

Sumo squat (Barbell)

- Remove the bar from the squat rack/Smith machine and support it across the top of your shoulders, at the back.
- Step your feet wider than shoulder-width apart with your feet turned outwards (make sure your knees are over your ankles and your toes are facing in the same direction as your knees).
- Lower the weight by bending your legs – aim to get your thighs parallel to the floor (but only lower within the confines of your flexibility).
- Extend your legs to stand back up. Keep your back flat throughout, core braced and chin up.

This version of the squat places more emphasis on your inner thighs and works the glutes and hamstrings differently.

TARGET MUSCLES AND FUNCTIONAL BENEFITS

- Quadriceps
- Glutes
- Hamstrings

⏱ 1:1 or 1:2

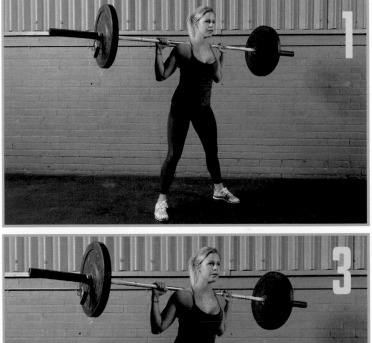

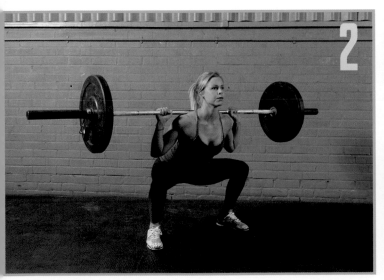

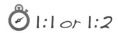 1:1 or 1:2

Front squat

- Remove the bar from the squat rack/Smith machine or clean it into position (see Clean).
- Stand upright with your feet just wider than shoulder-width. You should be supporting the weight on the front of your shoulders, with your fingers keeping it in place. In order to do this, your elbows must held high (don't let the bar make contact with your throat).
- Keep your head up and bend your legs to lower the weight. Don't lean forward as you do so.
- Extend your legs to stand back up. As with all squats, imagine that you are sitting and rising from a chair.

This version of the squat places more emphasis on your quads.

VARIATION

The front squat can be performed with kettlebells in much the same way, although you will need to learn how to clean them into position and then rack them – see kettlebell clean and press or snatch (page 144).

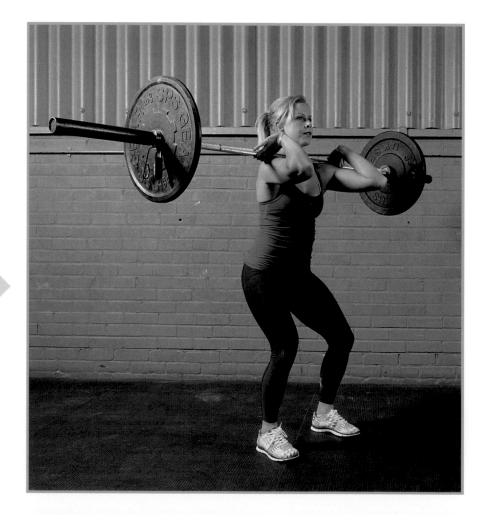

Offset lunge

- Hold a dumbbell at right angles to your body, at shoulder-height. Stand tall and strong.
- Take a large step into a lunge with the opposite leg to the arm holding the dumbbell.
- Push back through your heel to return to the start position. Brace your core throughout. As with all lunges, don't allow the knee of the lunging leg to pass to the sides or in front of your toes.

A great exercise for developing balance and stability.

TARGET MUSCLES AND FUNCTIONAL BENEFITS

- Glutes, quads and hamstrings when performing the lunge
- Core, arm and shoulder muscles to hold the weight in place

1:1

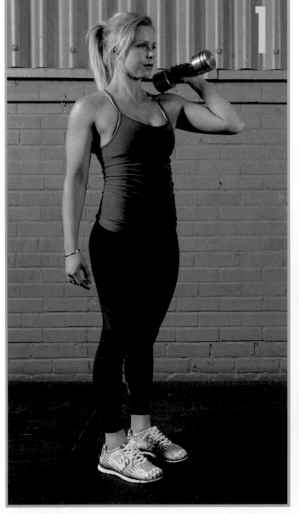

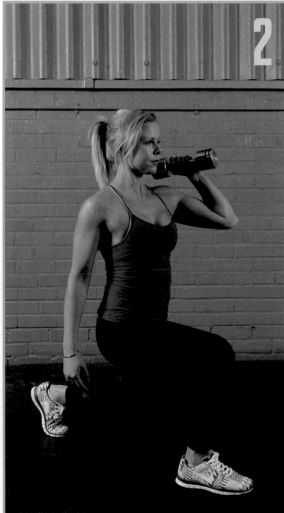

Kettlebell dead lift with reach

■ Hold a kettlebell at arm's length by your side, knuckles facing forward, and extend your other arm parallel to the floor.

■ Reach down towards the floor with the hand of the extended arm, allowing your torso to pivot forward, while bringing your leg (to the opposite side of the arm holding the kettlebell) up and straight.

■ Touch the floor with your free hand and the kettlebell before returning to the start position. Try to keep your back and standing leg straight throughout.

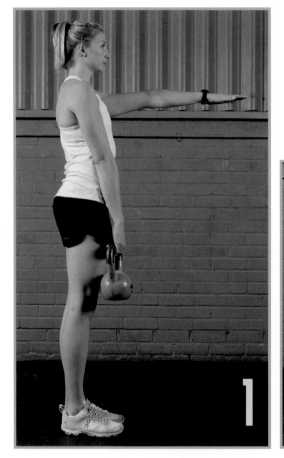

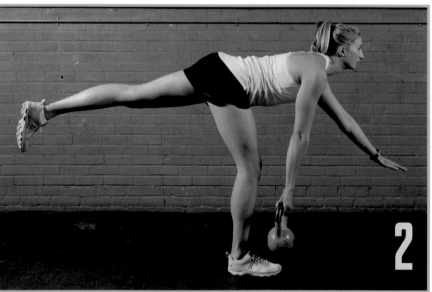

Kettlebell offset lunge

- Stand with your feet shoulder-width apart, holding the kettlebell at arm's length with a knuckles facing-away grip.
- Slowly curl the kettlebell up to your shoulder while keeping tension on your biceps muscle (you'll need good grip strength to do this).
- 'Fix' the kettlebell in position and then lunge forward on the opposite leg to the arm holding the kettlebell.
- Push back through the heel of your front foot and repeat. Use your opposite arm for balance by holding it parallel to the floor.

TARGET MUSCLES AND FUNCTIONAL BENEFITS

- Glutes
- Hamstrings
- Quads
- Core
- Shoulders
- Biceps
- Balance
- Coordination

⏱ 1:1 or 1:2

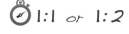 **TIP**

Start with a light weight and go heavier as you get stronger. This is a very challenging exercise initially.

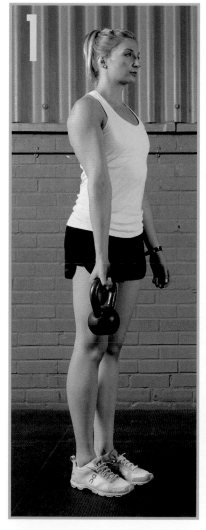

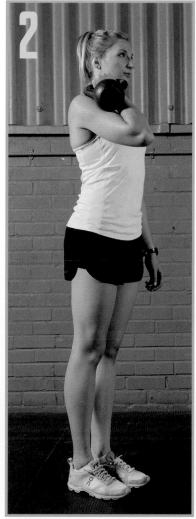

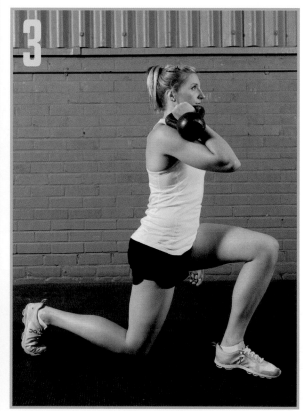

BOSU™

BOSU™ stands for 'both sides up' and this piece of training kit enables you to perform numerous exercises from a varying degree of instability. This means that your core muscles in particular need to work harder to control and centre the movement of the exercise you are performing.

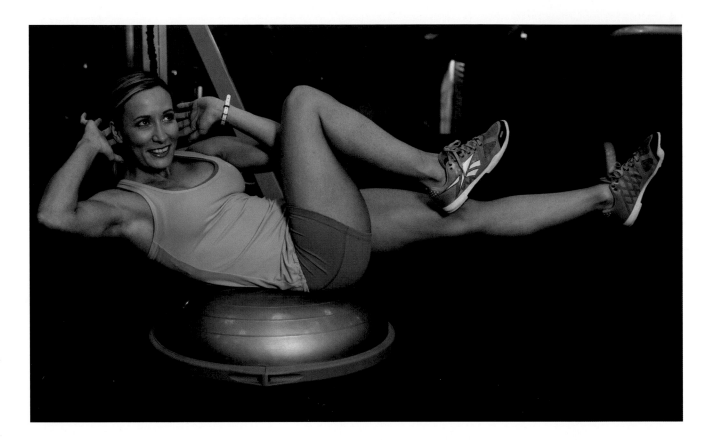

training

▶ Think for yourself!

You're an experienced resistance-trained woman now. By this stage – after reading and doing the exercises and workout programmes in this book – you will be very familiar with the majority of resistance training possibilities available to you. This, I hope, will allow you to develop your own programmes and adapt exercises accordingly. For example, if your gym does not have a suspension trainer or BOSU™, or it is not available at the time of your visit, you should be able to perform/select a different but similar exercise from those you'll find in this book (and any others that you are familiar with), knowing that they have a broadly similar function.

BOSU™ lunge (holding dumbbells)

- Place the BOSU™ in front of you, flat side down. Hold the dumbbells at arms' length by your sides.
- Take a large step back from the BOSU™ and then lunge onto it. Place your foot flat on the apex as you do so.
- Push back through your heel to return to the start position. Repeat on alternate legs.

Perform the exercise with control as the wobbly surface will create lateral forces, which you'll need to counteract.

⏱ 1:1
(but controlled)

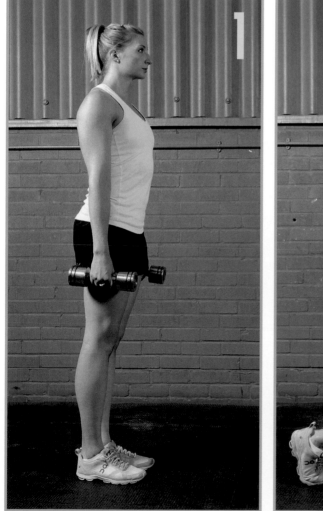

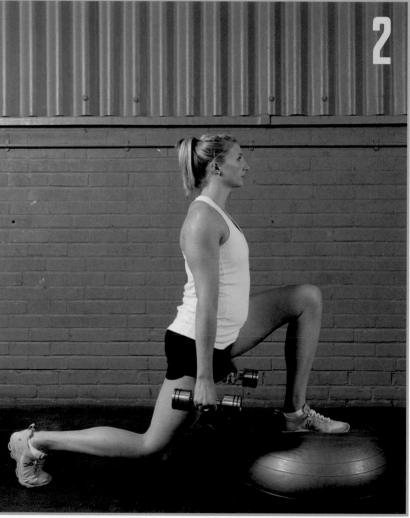

⏱ 1:1

BOSU™ squat jump

- Place the BOSU™ flat side down.
- Stand across the apex of the BOSU™ with your feet shoulder-width apart. Position your arms to aid your balance. Keep your back flat and your gaze focused straight ahead.
- Bend your knees and then jump into the air.
- Land on the BOSU™, reset yourself and repeat (you may need to reset yourself between jumps).

⊩ TIP

This is a dynamic exercise – progress sensibly. If you don't feel ready for it, replace with a squat (barbell or with dumbbells held at arms' length) or floor-based squat jump.

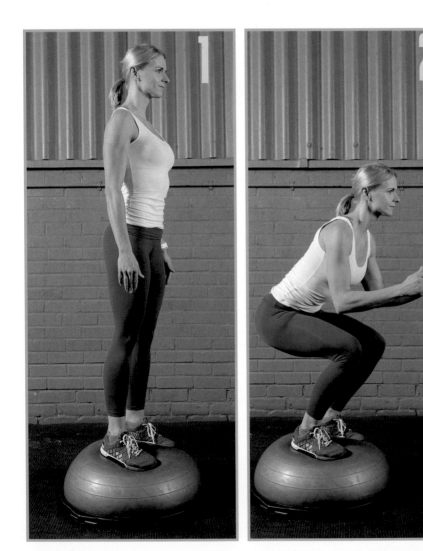

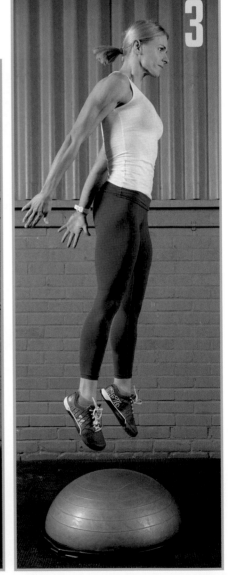

UPPER BODY EXERCISES

Bent over row

- With your toes under the bar and standing upright, bend your knees and take hold of it with a knuckles-on-top grip. Your hands should be outside your knees. Keep your shoulders over the bar.
- Straighten your legs slightly to lift the bar from the floor. The bar should be below your knees.
- Pull the bar up until it touches your lower chest. Your torso will be inclined forward. Brace your core throughout and maintain the natural curves of your spine.
- Extend your arms and repeat.

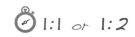

TARGET MUSCLES AND FUNCTIONAL BENEFITS

- Upper back
- Latissimus dorsi
- Triceps
- Lower back
- Glutes
- Hamstrings

🕐 1:1 or 1:2

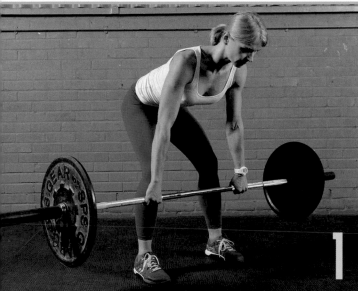

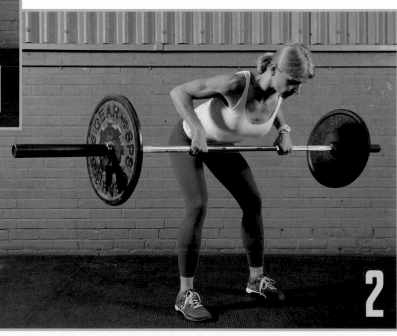

1:1 or 1:2

Prone row

■ Lie on an exercise
bench holding a
dumbbell in each
hand at arms' length
and below your
shoulders.

■ Pull the weights up
so that your upper
arms are parallel to
the floor.

■ Lower under control
and repeat.

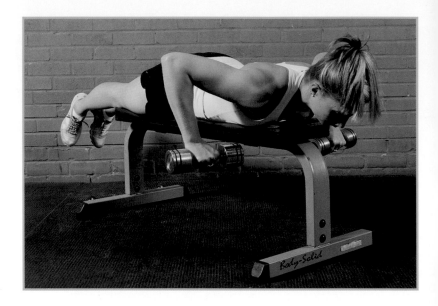

Press-up on bar

1:1

■ Load a barbell with large discs.
■ Assume a press-up position and take hold of the bar with an over-grasp shoulder-width grip.
■ Extend your arms and then lower under control so that your chest touches the bar.
   The bar will want to roll, requiring stabilisation. You supply this via your core and shoulders,
   which adds to the difficulty of the exercise.
■ Extend your arms and return to the start positon.

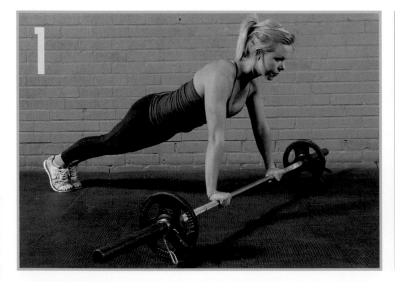

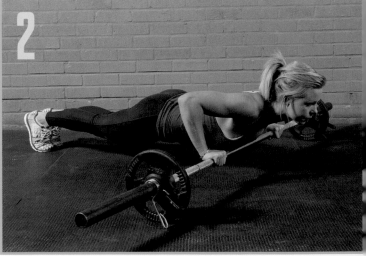

Suspension trainer press-up

- ■ Using a high anchor point, slide your feet into the straps from a prone position.
- ■ Place your hands in a standard press-up position, adjust your position and extend your arms.
- ■ Engage your core and lower your chest to the floor by bending your arms. Extend them to return to the start position.

1:1 or 1:2 or 2:2

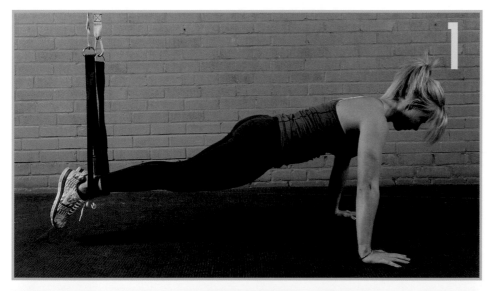

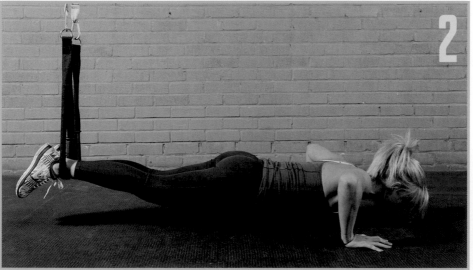

TARGET MUSCLES
AND FUNCTIONAL
BENEFITS

• Chest
• Core
• Front shoulders

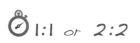

Suspension trainer chest press

- Position the anchor point overhead.
- Take hold of the handles (knuckles on top) and take a step back.
- Pull your shoulder blades down and activate your core.
- Lift one leg and hold the foot up behind you.
- Lean forwards, letting the straps move away from you, but keeping your arms extended and core braced. Bend your arms to initiate the movement and lower your chest towards the floor. When your arms are extended, your hands should be in line with your shoulders.
- Straighten your arms to return to the start position.

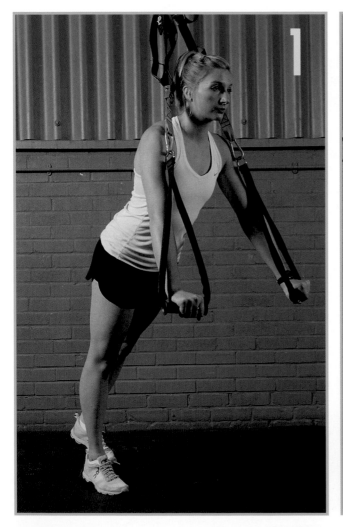

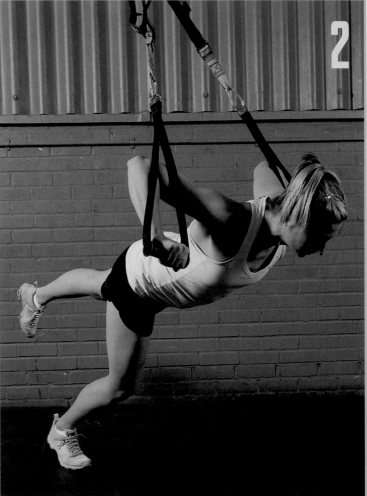

Suspension trainer reverse pull-up

- Using a high anchor point, lie on the floor and hold the suspension trainer handles with a knuckles-on-top grip and your arms extended.
- Bend your arms to pull your body higher and then extend your arms with control to return to the start position.

TARGET MUSCLES AND FUNCTIONAL BENEFITS

- Rear shoulders
- Upper back
- Core

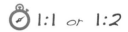

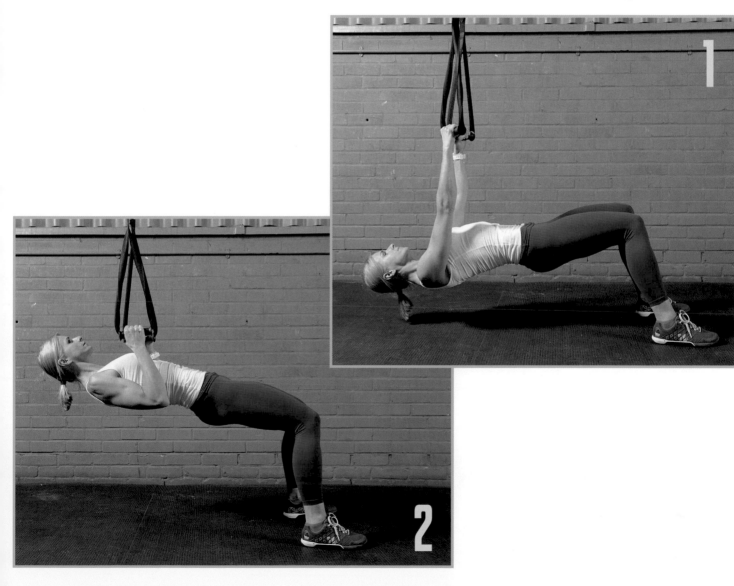

⏱ 1:1 (but
with control)

Kettlebell bottoms up single arm shoulder press

This is a tough exercise that really tests your grip strength, as well as your biceps and shoulder strength. Start with a light weight.

■ Assume a shoulder-width stance and hold one kettlebell by its handle with a knuckles facing back grip.

■ Slowly curl the kettlebell up to shoulder-height, keeping tension in your biceps. Rotate so your palm faces your body.

■ With the bottom (bell) of the kettlebell now facing up, press the kettlebell to full arm's extension.

■ Lower to shoulder-height and repeat.

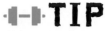

TIP

Make sure you focus on your breathing throughout – breathe in as you prepare and breathe out as you press the kettlebell up.

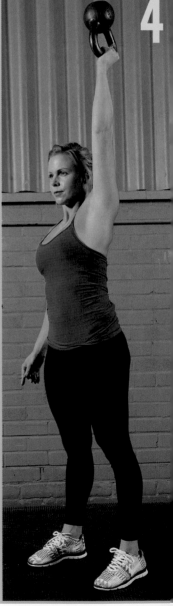

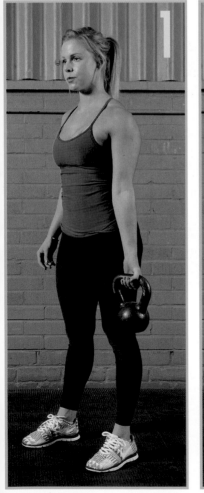

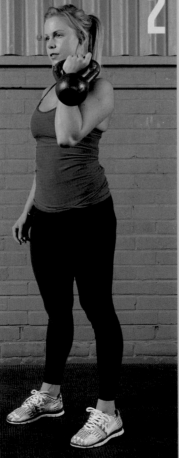

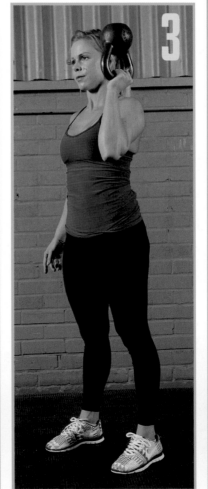

BOSU™ kneeling shoulder press

■ Kneel on the curved side of the BOSU™, holding a dumbbell in each hand at arms' length.
■ Stabilise yourself – which will require core activation – and then press the dumbbells to overhead.
■ Pause and then lower under control.

A great exercise for developing a toned stomach and arms.

 1:1

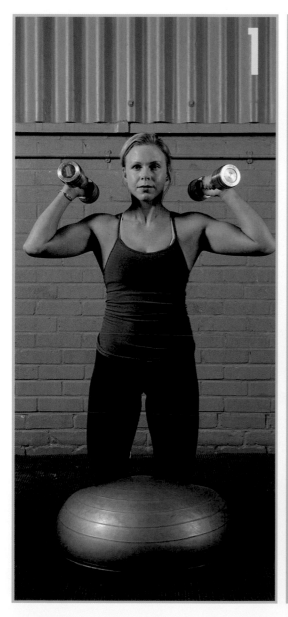

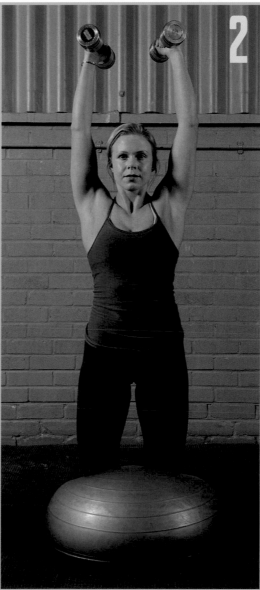

⏱ 1:1

BOSU™ Spiderman

You have to really work your core to stabilise throughout this move as the BOSU™ will tilt from side-to-side.

■ Position the BOSU™ so that the flat side is up. Place your hands centrally and to the edges of the BOSU™ so that your arms are about shoulder-width apart. With your legs extended and your feet about hip-width apart, make sure your body is in a straight line.

■ Perform a press-up and, as you lower, bring one of your knees in towards the elbow on the same side.

■ Push up and simultaneously extend your leg to the start position.

■ Repeat with the other leg.

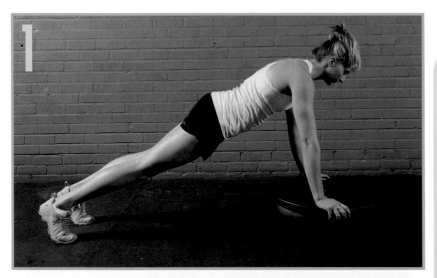

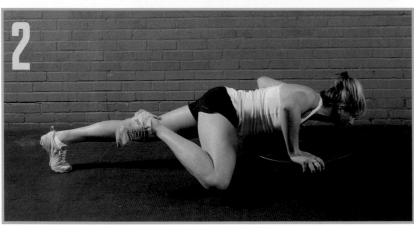

training equipment

Suspension Trainers

All suspension trainer exercises target the core. Indeed, one of the great claims of suspension training is the unique way that it stresses our back, stomach and sides. Because of the way the suspension trainer generates forces (rotational and linear), certain exercises mean that the core has to adjust, control and move with the exercise in different and, on occasion, more demanding ways than if you were performing a similar exercise without suspension.

Studies have shown that muscle activation is higher when suspension training compared to performing the same activities without it.

CORE EXERCISES

TARGET MUSCLES
AND FUNCTIONAL
BENEFITS

- Core
- Shoulders

Suspension trainer plank

- Use a high anchor point. Slip your feet into the stirrups and get into a plank position. Keep your hands under your shoulders and align the back of your head, shoulders, bottom and heels.
- Hold for a designated time and remember to breathe throughout!

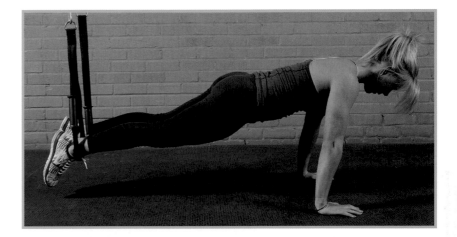

Suspension trainer in and out

- Assume a similar position to the previous exercise; however, this time pull both knees in towards your chest and then push them away to the starting position.

⏱ 1:1

TARGET MUSCLES
AND FUNCTIONAL
BENEFITS

- Hip flexors
- Core
- Shoulders

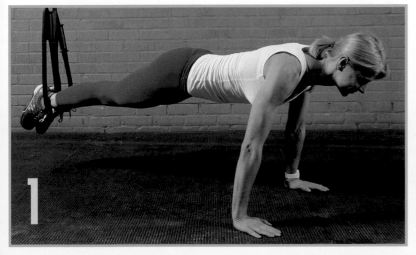

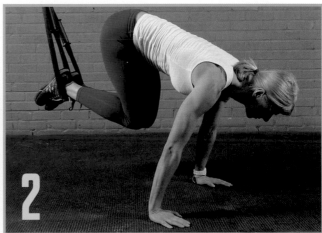

TARGET MUSCLES AND FUNCTIONAL BENEFITS

- Hip flexors
- Core
- Shoulders

⏱ 1:1

Suspension trainer diagonal reverse crunch

■ Assume the same starting position as for a plank.
■ Pull your knees into your chest and twist your torso right and left before extending your knees back to the start position – this is one rep.

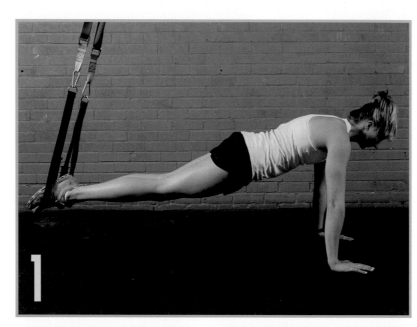

This exercise will really target your obliques and help to create a toned and slimmer abdomen.

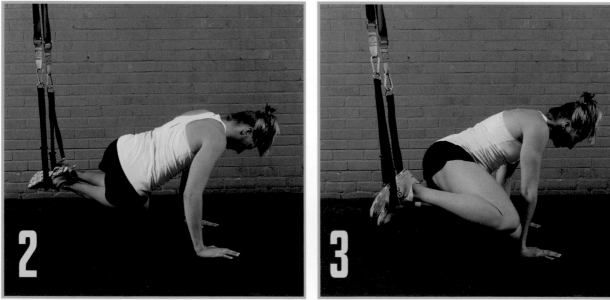

Suspension trainer atomic press-up

- Assume a similar position to the previous three exercises.
- Pull your knees into your chest and then extend your legs, as with the In and Out.
  Pause the movement – you'll be in a plank position, now perform a press-up.
- Pull your knees into your chest to start the next repeat and continue as before.

1:1

This exercise has a very high metabolic cost and is a very difficult move.

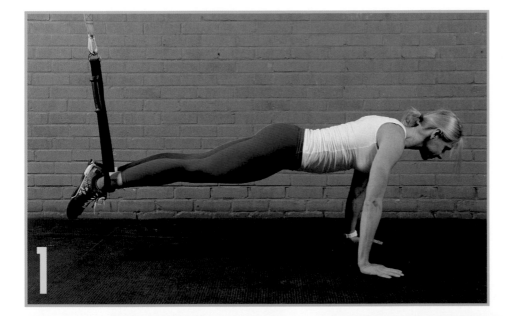

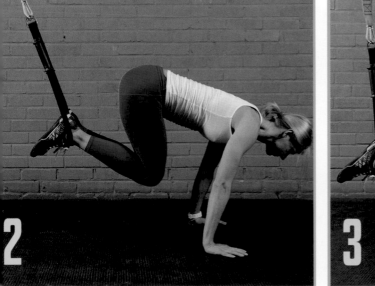

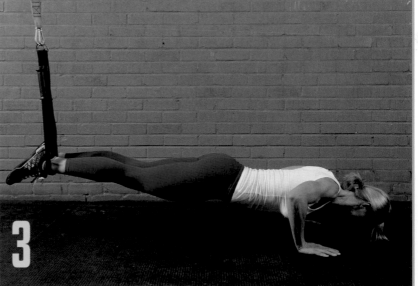

Kettlebell side plank

■ Assume a side plank position but place one leg over the other (do not stack your feet one on top of the other as you would with a standard side plank). Doing it this way will also target your glutes.

■ Lift the kettlebell into position and hold at arm's length for a designated time.

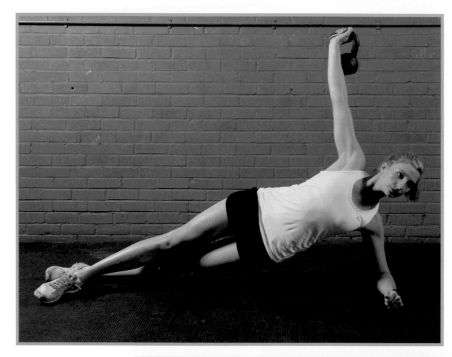

ADVANCED VARIATION
Perform the exercise as described above, but this time lift your upper leg up as well and hold.

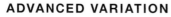

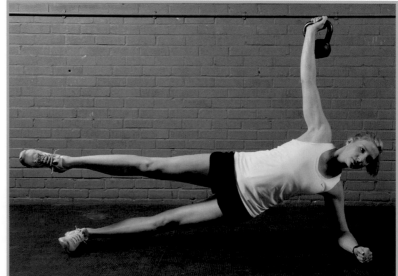

BOSU™ bicycle

- Place the BOSU™ flat side down and position yourself so that your bottom and lower back are on the apex of the curved side.
- Extend one leg and lean back.
- Simultaneously pull the extended leg into and across your body to the opposite shoulder as you bring your trunk forward.
- Push the leg away from you as you lean back.
- Repeat, reversing the movement. Keep your hands by your ears throughout and keep the non-working leg straight.

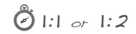

TARGET MUSCLES AND FUNCTIONAL BENEFITS

- Core, particularly obliques and hip flexors

⏱ 1:1 or 1:2

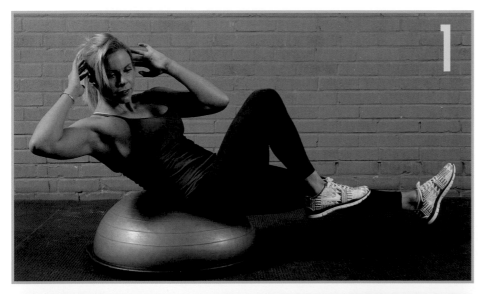

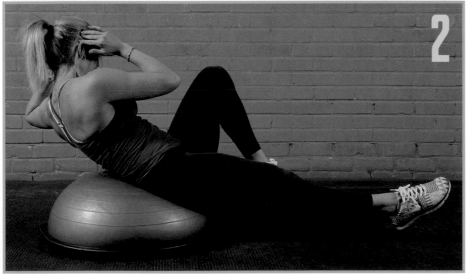

This is a great shaper and strength-builder for your lower abs and obliques.

ALL BODY EXERCISES

TARGET MUSCLES AND FUNCTIONAL BENEFITS

- Chest
- Shoulders
- Glutes
- Hamstrings
- Quads
- Calves

⏱ 1:2
(control the downward path)

Clean

- Squat down and take hold of the bar with your knuckles facing forwards and hands just wider than shoulder-width apart. Keep your heels on the floor, your arms extended and your head up. Maintain the natural curves of your spine and brace your core.
- Drive your legs up to lift the bar from the floor, keeping your shoulders over it.
- Extend up onto your toes, keeping the bar in close to your body.
- As the bar approaches hip level, drive your hips forwards and pull on the bar with your arms. As you do this, bend your knees to drop below the bar, letting the bar go from below your wrists to over them.
- Straighten your legs.
- To complete the movement, 'catch' the bar in a racked position on the front of your shoulders (in a similar position to the front squat).
- Keeping your back flat, control the bar down to the floor, bending your knees and folding forwards, first to your thighs and then to the floor.

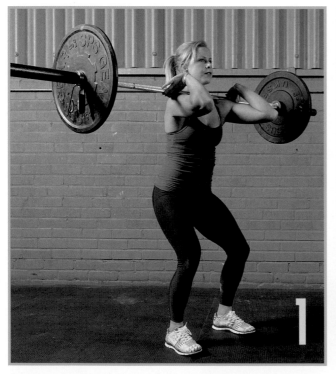

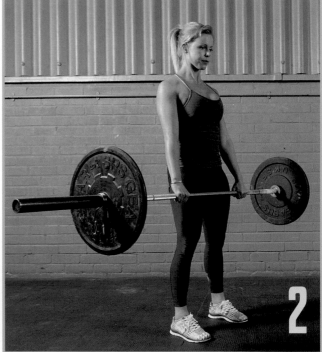

Single arm kettlebell swing

- Start the exercise as indicated, pulling the kettlebell in, before swinging it forward and up.
- Bend your knees and drive your hips forward to start to propel the weight up. Keep your core braced throughout.
- When your hips are extended, your torso upright and the kettlebell near to shoulder-level, let it drop back down and through your legs. Move with the fall of the kettlebell and let your bottom move backwards and torso incline forwards.
- As the momentum of the weight begins to stall and go in the other direction, 'snap' your hips to extend them to impart more momentum onto the kettlebell to drive it forwards and up again. You do not use your arms/shoulders to lift the weight – rather it is driven up from the action of your hips and glutes. Use your non-working arm for balance.

TARGET MUSCLES AND FUNCTIONAL BENEFITS

- Quads
- Hamstrings
- Glutes
- Core
- Shoulders

⏱ 1:1

The swing is a great exercise for shaping your glutes as the drive from the exercise comes primarily from here and the hips.

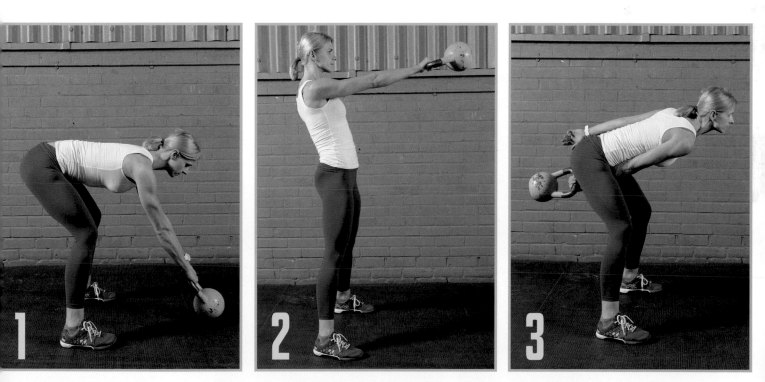

▶ **VARIATION**
The exercise can also be performed with both hands gripping the kettlebell's handles – the two-handed swing.

TARGET MUSCLES AND FUNCTIONAL BENEFITS

- Glutes
- Hamstrings
- Quads
- Core
- Chest
- Shoulders

1:1

Kettlebell clean

This is a very dynamic exercise and the unilateral action will mean that your core has to stabilise the entire movement – spend time mastering correct technique before progressing to using a heavier kettlebell.

- As with the swing, take hold of the kettlebell in one hand with your knuckles facing away from you.
- Bend your legs and then extend them to start to propel the weight up, this time keeping your arm long and close in to your body.
- As the weight nears your hips drive them forward, extend onto your toes and pull on the kettlebell with your arm. At the same time, bend your knees to drop below the ascending kettlebell and rotate your wrist, so that the kettlebell flips over to the back of your wrist.
- Straighten your legs – the kettlebell should be racked in front of your shoulder.
- Control the path of the kettlebell back to the start position by moving with it.

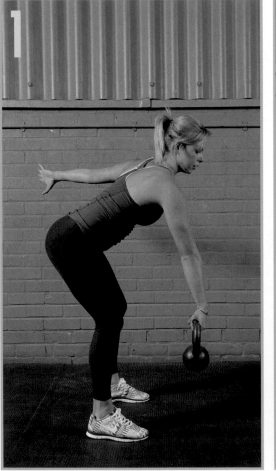
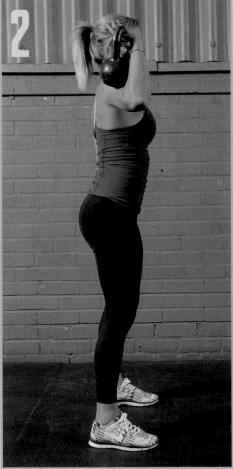

VARIATION
The exercise can also be performed with two kettlebells, adding to the coordination and strength requirements of the exercise.

Kettlebell clean and press

- Clean the kettlebell into the racked position as described previously in the clean, pause for a brief moment, then 'punch' your arm straight up to press the kettlebell to arm's length.
- Lower under control back to the racked position and control the path of the kettlebell back to the start position.

TARGET MUSCLES AND FUNCTIONAL BENEFITS

- Glutes
- Hamstrings
- Quads
- Core
- Chest
- Shoulders

 1:1

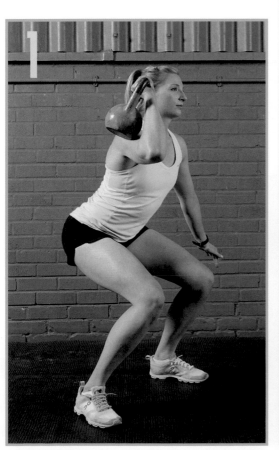

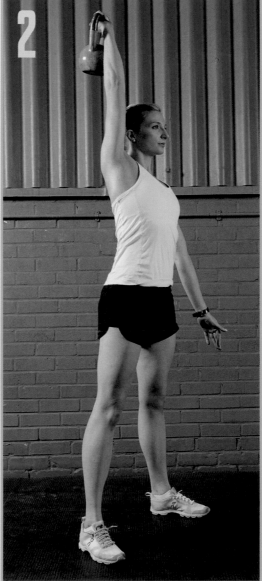

⏱ 1:1

Kettlebell snatch

This is another very dynamic, all body, high metabolic cost kettlebell exercise.

■ This exercise requires you to lift one kettlebell dynamically and continuously from a swing to overhead.

■ As with the clean, extend your thighs and dynamically 'snap' your hips to power up the kettlebell. Control the arc of the weight and keep it close to your body, unlike with the swing.

■ When the weight is around waist height, pull your elbow up and to the outside of your torso, then dynamically punch 'through' the kettlebell and fully extend your arm and body as you do so. It should flip over and end on the back of your wrist. Aim for your biceps to be close to your ear at the top of the movement.

■ Control the weight on the way down and, when transitioning into another rep, push your bottom back when the bell is around waist height. This puts your glutes and hamstrings in the ideal position to launch the bell into another rep.

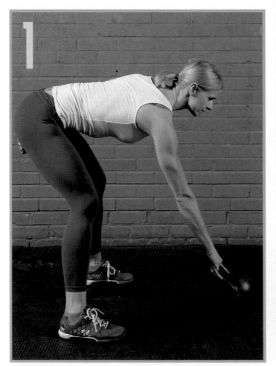

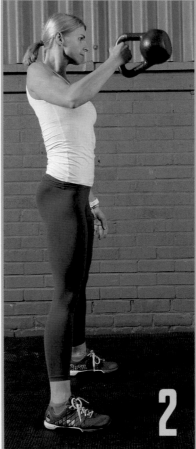

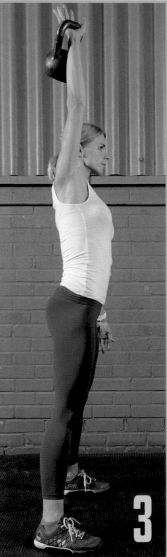

BOSU™ burpee

- Take hold of the BOSU™ at its sides and lift it to arms' length in front of your chest, with the flat side facing you.
- Bend your knees and extend your arms to place the BOSU™ on the floor in front of you.
- With your hands evenly spaced near the centre edges, jump your back feet into a plank position.
- Perform a press-up and then jump your legs in while simultaneously lifting the BOSU™ overhead.
- Bring the BOSU™ back to the start position and repeat.

TARGET MUSCLES AND FUNCTIONAL BENEFITS

- Glutes
- Hamstrings
- Quads
- Chest
- Biceps
- Triceps
- Shoulders
- Core

 VARIATION
Those new to this exercise can omit the press-up.

1:1

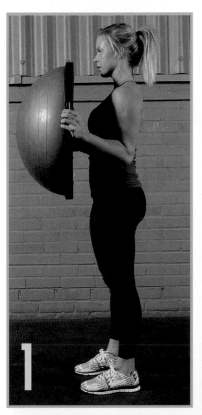

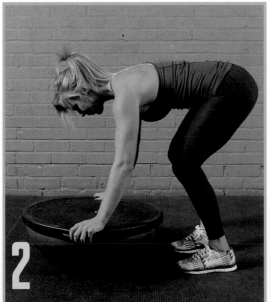

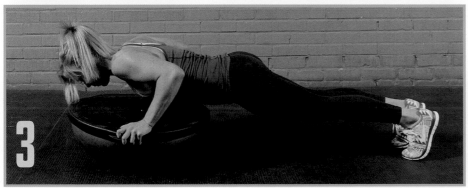

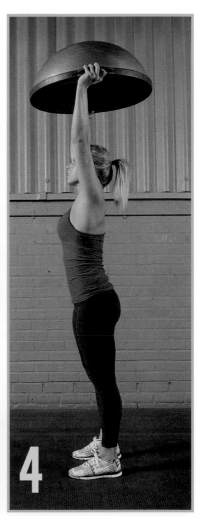

🕐 1:1

This is a tough exercise that brings into play virtually every muscle in your body.

BOSU™ single leg raise and dumbbell chest press

■ Lie on the floor with a dumbbell in one hand over your same-side shoulder.

■ Place the heel of one extended leg on top of the BOSU™ and lift the other. As you do this, press the heel of the extended leg into the BOSU™ to lift your hips.

■ Holding this position, perform a designated number of reps of shoulder presses.

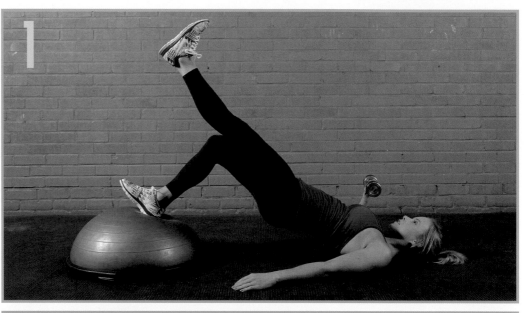

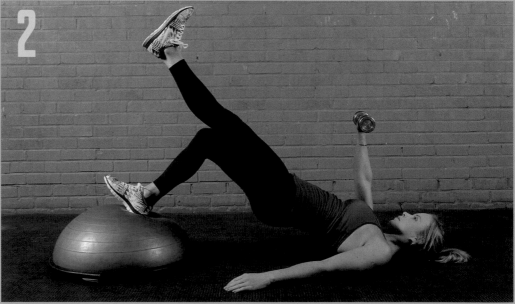

GETTING STRONGER, FIRMER AND FITTER

The workouts that follow will take your resistance training to the next level, involving new exercises, new equipment and new training systems. You'll see that I stress the need to progress safely and only once you have learned correct exercise technique. The first two weeks of the programme therefore include technique sessions to enable you to learn the majority of the new exercises. If, as in the previous phase, you have any doubts about your ability to perform any of the exercises safely, contact a personal trainer or fitness professional for further advice. And again you can change some of the exercises for similar alternatives if you don't feel ready for certain ones or if equipment is limited.

A note on stretching

Too much stretching before a workout can actually be counterproductive when it comes to getting the most out of your resistance training. Muscles need to be reactive and able to exert force. Holding stretches for more than 10 seconds in particular can reduce muscles' ability to express force. Hence, you should perform functional movements in your warm-ups, such as marching on the spot, arm swings, heel raises and so on. These should be completed after 5 minutes or so of CV work, preferably jogging. These exercises will prepare your muscles and joints much more specifically for the work that will follow.

The time to stretch

There is value in stretching. You can perform some light stretches after your workouts – but tired muscles that have been worked hard should not be overstretched. It's best to work on what's called 'developmental' stretches away from your resistance workouts. So, you could stretch on your days off or in the evenings. This is the time when you can push further into your stretches in an attempt to increase your range of movement. Select stretches for all body parts and hold for 15–20 seconds. **Note:** Although you may not initially appreciate it, resistance training can actually develop flexibility. The kettlebell swing, for example will develop/maintain shoulder, lower back and hip range of movement.

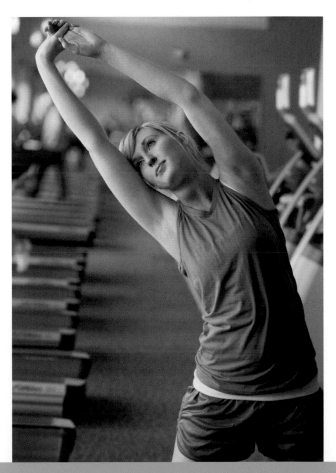

RATE OF PRECEIVED EXERTION FOR THE SECOND 12-WEEK WORKOUT PHASE

In this phase, emphasis is placed on the development of strength and creating the optimum conditions for muscles to increase the lean mass of your body and therefore improve its calorie burning potential. RPEs – unlike in the first 12 weeks of the programme – are less relevant for some of the workouts. This is because of the different emphasis – they are often concerned with the development of strength and rest periods need to be long to enable a full-on commitment to the lifts. RPEs are therefore only provided for some of the sessions where this suits.

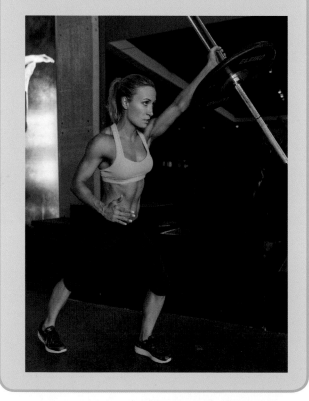

▶ A guide to what weight to lift

In the workout tables in this chapter, as in the last one, you'll see that exercises have been given a suggested weight to use as designated, for example, medium weight, heavy weight and so on. These align to the rep ranges suggested below. Note that these are guidelines to give you an idea of what weight you should be lifting each workout. They require the last reps in each set to be difficult to complete but with good form. In reality, they will vary slightly between individuals because of previous weight training familiarity (exercises and exercise system, for example) and motivation.

Weight to lift	Rep Range	Approx % of 1RM
Light weight	10–20 plus	20–50%
Light/medium weight	8–12	50–60%
Medium weight	6–10	60–70%
Medium/heavy weight	4–8	70–80%
Heavy weight	3–6	80–90%
Heavy/very heavy weight	1–3	90–100%

THE TRAINING PROGRAMME WEEKS 13-24

☎ Weeks 13-16 Resisting - Advanced 1

<table>
<tr><th colspan="2">WEEK
TRAINING
SYSTEM</th><th>EXERCISES AND RPE
(Where relevant)</th><th>OTHER COMMENTS</th></tr>
<tr><td>1</td><td>SS Weights
Barbell,
suspension
trainer,
kettlebells,
Swiss ball</td><td>• Barbell clean; Barbell front squat 3 x 6–8;
Suspension trainer plank 3 x 30sec; Kettlebell bottoms up shoulder press 3 x 8 L&R; Swiss ball hamstring curls 3 x 30sec
• Take as much recovery as you need to complete the exercises and learn their technique</td><td>• The aim of this session and others this week is to familiarise you with new exercises and their technique. Spend time mastering them and lifting a sensible, light weight if you have little or no experience of them. With more experience, venture to medium weight territory, where appropriate. Familiar exercises are included from the first 12 weeks of the programme.</td></tr>
<tr><td>2</td><td>SS Kettlebells
and BOSU™</td><td>• Kettlebells: Single leg dead lift with reach 3 x 8 (L&R); Two-handed swing 3 x 8; Single arm clean 3 x 6 (L&R)
• Take 40sec between each exercise and perform a set of each and then a set of the next – going round the exercises in circuit style
• All with light weight
• BOSU™: Bicycle crunch 3 x 12 (one rep equals a movement to both sides, therefore your set will comprise 24 movements); Forward lunge 3 x 10 (L&R)
• Take as much recovery as you need to complete the exercises and learn technique</td><td>• Again, this session is all about learning how to do the exercises. You should take it very easily if you are not familiar with the new ones. Use a light weight.</td></tr>
<tr><td>3</td><td>CV
Running</td><td>• Easy 20min run at RPE 2–4</td><td>• This is a recovery session so stick to the RPE.</td></tr>
<tr><td>4</td><td>SS
Weights – all
kettlebells</td><td>• Snatch 3 x 6 (L&R); Clean and press 3 x 5 (L&R); Offset lunge 3 x 8 (L&R); Side plank 3 x 15sec (L&R); Kettlebell single leg dead lift with reach 3 x 6 (L&R)
• Take 40sec between each exercise and perform a set of each exercise and then a set of the next – going round the exercises in circuit style
• All with light weight
• Take as much recovery as you need to complete the exercises and learn technique</td><td>• Again, it's about learning the new exercises, although this workout will still have a high metabolic cost.</td></tr>
</table>

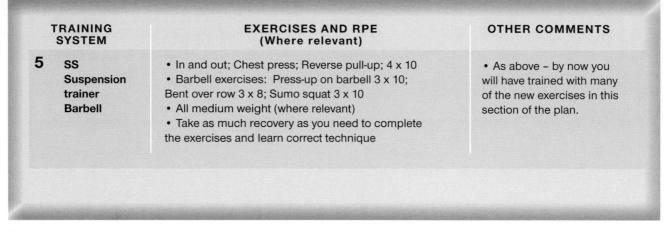

TRAINING SYSTEM	EXERCISES AND RPE (Where relevant)	OTHER COMMENTS
5 **SS** **Suspension trainer** **Barbell**	• In and out; Chest press; Reverse pull-up; 4 x 10 • Barbell exercises: Press-up on barbell 3 x 10; Bent over row 3 x 8; Sumo squat 3 x 10 • All medium weight (where relevant) • Take as much recovery as you need to complete the exercises and learn correct technique	• As above – by now you will have trained with many of the new exercises in this section of the plan.

This will be a real learning week (and so too will be the next), as you familiarise your mind and body with an array of new exercises. Many are more dynamic than those in the first 12 weeks of the programme – but you should be conditioned enough to handle them by now. Remember to take your time to learn proper technique for each and use a very light weight, where relevant. Don't feel the need to rush – you will still be getting a training benefit. And once you have mastered correct technique there'll be plenty more workouts to tackle greater resistances in this programme and beyond.

WEEK 14

TRAINING SYSTEM	EXERCISES AND RPE (Where relevant)	OTHER COMMENTS
1 **SS Weights** **Barbell,** **suspension** **trainer,** **kettlebells,** **Swiss ball**	• Barbell clean; Barbell squat; 3 x 8 light to medium weight; Barbell bent over row 3 x 8 light weight; Suspension trainer press-up 3 x 12; Kettlebell bottoms up shoulder press; 3 x 8 L&R light to medium weight; Swiss ball hamstring curl 3 x 30sec • Take as much recovery as you need to complete the exercises and learn technique	• This workout develops the similar one last week. A couple of new exercises are added and the idea is that you begin to lift slightly heavier weights than last week, where applicable. • It's important that you keep a training diary and log what you lift each session.
2 **SS Weights:** **Kettlebells** **and BOSU™**	• Kettlebells: Single leg dead lift with reach 3 x 8 (L&R); Two-handed swing 3 x 8; Single arm clean 3 x 8 (L&R) • Take 30sec between each exercise and perform a set of each exercise and then a set of the next – going round the exercises in circuit style • 5min recovery • BOSU™: Bicycle; Single leg lift with chest press 3 x 10 (L&R); Spiderman 3 x 12; Forward lunge 3 x 10 (L&R) • 30sec between exercises	• Again, up the weights possibly to a medium intensity one, should you feel confident enough. If you do so, the last couple of reps in each set should feel difficult.

TRAINING SYSTEM	EXERCISES AND RPE (Where relevant)	OTHER COMMENTS
3 CV Running	• Easy 20min run at RPE 2–4	• This is a recovery session so stick to the RPE.
4 SS Kettlebell dominant all-body workout High metabolic cost SS Body weight abs circuit	• Snatch 3 x 8 (L&R); Clean (3 x 8 L&R), Offset lunge (3 x 10 L&R); Side plank (3 x 20sec L&R); Kettlebell single leg dead lift with reach 3 x 8 (L&R); Single arm swing 3 x 8 (L&R) • Take 40sec between each exercise and perform a set of each and then a set of the next – going round the exercises in circuit style • 5min recovery • Body weight – abs circuit: Toe tap; Plank with leg lift; Glute bridge 3 x 20sec – take 10sec recovery between each exercise	• Use a light weight for the kettlebell exercises.
5 SuS Barbell SS Suspension trainer	• Barbell (unless otherwise indicated) • SuS 1: Offset lunge (dumbbell) 3 x 10 (L&R) and Sumo squat 3 x 10 light weight • SuS 2: Clean (light/medium weight) and Press-up on bar 3 x 10 • SuS 3: Prone row light weight dumbbells and Dead lift 3 x 10 medium weight • 5min recovery • Suspension trainer: Atomic press-up; Reverse pull-up 3 x 10 • Take 30sec between each exercise (longer if you need it)	• Remember that for the supersets you should perform a set of one exercise in the pair and then immediately follow it with the next. Then rest for 2min and complete the next superset. Rest a further 2min between each superset pairing.

By the end of this week, you will have used most of the new exercises in this chapter's plans. The emphasis is still on learning technique, although the intensity of some of the workouts has increased from last week's.

ADAPT AND PROGRESS WHEN READY. BE SENSIBLE!

I'd really hope that by now, should your gym not have the necessary items of equipment referenced in the workout tables and/or you don't yet feel ready for the workouts or exercises, you will be able to select a replacement that will have a broadly similar effect. For example, you could replace the front squat with the single leg squat (see page 55) or the Bulgarian split squat. Likewise, the suspension trainer plank could be replaced with the plank and leg lift (see page 76).

	TRAINING SYSTEM	EXERCISES AND RPE (Where relevant)	OTHER COMMENTS
1	**SuS and SS Weights Barbell, kettlebells, Swiss ball**	• Barbell • SuS 1: Squat and Front squat 3 x 5 medium weight • SuS 2: Dead lift and Bent over row 3 x 8 medium weight • Prone row (dumbbells) 3 x 8 medium weight • Kettlebell bottoms up shoulder press 3 x 12 (L&R) light to medium weight • Swiss ball hamstring curls 3 x 30sec	• The supersets – now with a consistently heavier weight – will really create the best conditions for your body to respond positively by releasing health and vitality hormones. • The second superset of dead lifts and bent over rows will really target your glutes and hamstrings to shape a great-looking bottom.
2	**SS Kettlebell dominant all-body workout High metabolic cost SS BOSU™ blast**	• Single leg dead lift with reach 3 x 8 (L&R); Two-handed swing 3 x 8; Snatch 3 x 8 (L&R); Offset lunge 3 x 10 (L&R); Bottoms up shoulder press 3 x 10 (L&R) – all light/medium weight • Take 30sec between each exercise and perform a set of each and then a set of the next – going round the exercises in circuit style • 10min recovery • BOSU™ Burpee; BOSU™ Jump squat 3 x 12 • Take 30secs between exercises	• An increase in reps will make the session more demanding, as will the dynamic BOSU exercises.
3	**P Weights Body weight abs circuit**	• Barbell: Clean; Squat; Bent over row • 10 x light weight • 6 x medium weight • 4 x 3 medium/heavy weight • 5 min recovery • Body weight – abs circuit: Russian twist; Plank with leg lift (alternate left/right leg lifts); Feet elevated crunch • 3 x 20sec – take 10sec recovery between each exercise	• Your first pyramid session in this part of the plan. Take as much time as you need between sets to give yourself the best possible chance of completing the exercises. Use squat racks for the front squat (the beauty of this exercise is that you can drop the bar, should you need to).

This is a lighter intensity week in terms of the number of workouts you have to perform – just three (and make sure you have at least a day between each). However, the intensity of each is high and your body will appreciate the recovery – remember it's in the time when you are not training that it repairs and all the positive gains occur.

A training programme needs to vary its intensity in order to avoid stagnation and allow for continued progression and enthusiasm.

	TRAINING SYSTEM	EXERCISES AND RPE (Where relevant)	OTHER COMMENTS
1	SS Weights SS Barbell and Suspension trainer circuit	• Barbell: Clean; Front squat; 3 x 8 medium/heavy weight • Bent over row 3 x 12 medium weight • 5min recovery • Suspension trainer: Plank 3 x 40sec hold; Reverse pull-up 3 x 12; Diagonal reverse crunch 3 x 12 • Take 30sec between exercises	• Again, this workout develops on last week's one. You should be lifting progressively heavier weights compared to last week, where applicable. • A couple of new suspension exercises are also added. • The suspension trainer reverse pull-up is great for upper body strength.
2	SS Kettlebell dominant all-body workout High metabolic cost SS BOSU™ blast	• Single arm clean 3 x 10 (L&R); Single leg dead lift with reach 3 x 8 (L&R); One-handed swing 3 x 10 (L&R); Offset lunge 3 x 10 (L&R); Bottoms up shoulder press 3 x 10 (L&R) – all light/medium weight. • Take 30sec between each exercise and perform a set of each exercise and then a set of the next – going round the exercises in circuit style • 5min recovery • BOSU™: Forward lunge 3 x 12 (L&R); Burpee 3 x 12; Jump squat 3 x 12. • Take 30sec between exercises	• The last couple of reps in each set should feel difficult, but you must be in control of the exercises due to their dynamic nature. • Another 2 reps have been added to each exercise over last week's workout.
3	CV Sprints	• 10 x 10sec sprints at RPE 5–7/8 • 2min walk recovery at RPE 2–4	• Sprinting targets all your body's muscles and is a great way to burn calories and develop lean muscle. Warm up thoroughly before this session. • As before (see Weeks 1–12 workout programme), you could do a similar session on an exercise bike.
4	SuS Barbell Suspension trainer SS	• Barbell (unless otherwise indicated) • SuS 1: Offset lunge (dumbbell) 3 x 10 medium weight and Sumo squat 3 x 8 medium weight • SuS 2: Clean 3 x 10 (medium weight) and Press-up on bar 3 x 12 • SuS 3: Prone row (light weight) and Dead lift 3 x 10 (medium weight) • 5min recovery • Suspension trainer: Atomic press-up; Reverse pull up 3 x 10; Plank 30sec hold • Take 30sec between each exercise.	• Increase your weights if you can – but sensibly, within the suggested target weight. • Remember that for the supersets you should perform a set of one exercise and immediately follow it with the next in the pair. Then rest for 2min and complete the next superset.

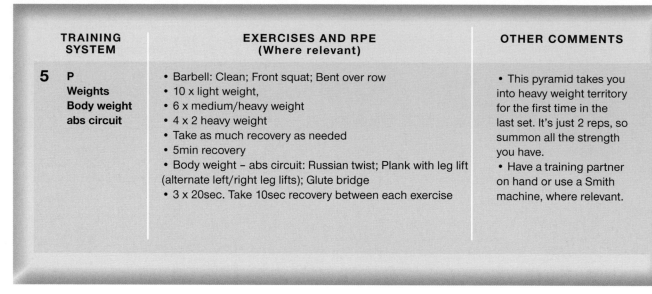

TRAINING SYSTEM	EXERCISES AND RPE (Where relevant)	OTHER COMMENTS
5 P Weights Body weight abs circuit	• Barbell: Clean; Front squat; Bent over row • 10 x light weight, • 6 x medium/heavy weight • 4 x 2 heavy weight • Take as much recovery as needed • 5min recovery • Body weight – abs circuit: Russian twist; Plank with leg lift (alternate left/right leg lifts); Glute bridge • 3 x 20sec. Take 10sec recovery between each exercise	• This pyramid takes you into heavy weight territory for the first time in the last set. It's just 2 reps, so summon all the strength you have. • Have a training partner on hand or use a Smith machine, where relevant.

This is a tougher week following the previous easier one. By now, you should really be confident in your lifting ability and in your new found strength!

Weeks 17–20   Resisting - Advanced 2

This block of training builds on the last and there's much more of an emphasis on pushing your body that bit harder, as by now you should be able to perform the majority of the exercises with good technique and you'll have developed a very good level of strength. The training systems giant sets (GS) and drop sets (DS) are introduced. Here's a reminder of what they entail:

Drop sets: Start with a heavy load on the bar – for example, a medium/heavy weight, around 75 per cent of 1RM – and complete as many reps as possible. Weight is then taken off the bar and as many reps as possible are completed again immediately. This process continues for a designated number of sets or until potentially there is no weight left on the bar. This obviously makes for a very tough session and one that requires considerable willpower. It can also be done with dumbbells.

Giant sets: This training system is similar to supersets but involves any number of sets of exercises joined together, one after the other. Giant sets can focus on a body part or include exercises that utilize different muscular actions, or they can be random. As with superset pairs, you move straight from one exercise in the giant set to the next and so on and then, after completing all, you take a rest and perform the same giant set again or move on to another.

17

	TRAINING SYSTEM	EXERCISES AND RPE (Where relevant)	OTHER COMMENTS
1	**SS** **Weights** **SS** **Barbell and Suspension trainer circuit**	• Barbell: Clean; Front squat; 4 x 8 medium weight; Bent over row 4 x 10 light–medium weight • Take as much rest as necessary between sets • 5min recovery • Suspension trainer: Plank 4 x 40sec hold; Reverse pull-up 4 x 12; Atomic press-up 4 x 12 • Take 40sec between exercises	• Reps are increased on all exercises from previous similar workouts.
2	**GS** **Kettlebells** **Core exercise**	• GS 1: Two-handed swing x 10; One-hand swing (L&R) x 10; Single arm clean x 10 (L&R) x 3 (take 60sec at the end of each GS) • 5min recovery • GS 2: Racked front squat x 20; Clean and press x 10 (L&R); Offset lunge x 10 (L&R) x 3 (take 60sec at the end of each GS) Use light to medium weight • 5min recovery • Core exercise: Side plank advanced option 3 x 20sec (L&R) • 30sec recovery between sets	• The beauty of kettlebells is that they can produce a dynamic, fluent and high metabolic cost workout – with the ability to transition between movements virtually seamlessly. Each giant set will comprise 50 movements (accounting for movements to both sides of your body), each performed three times. This is a tough workout – be warned.
3	**CV** **Sprints**	• 10 x 10sec sprints at RPE 7/8 • 2min walk recovery at RPE 2–4 • As usual, make sure you warm up thoroughly	• You could replace this session with stadium step sprints, taking one or two at a time, or do the bike option as previously suggested if you wanted a change.
4	**P** **Weights** **SS** **Body weight abs circuit**	• Barbell (unless otherwise indicated): Clean; Squat; Prone row (dumbbell) • 10 x light weight • 8 x medium weight • 3 x 4 heavy weight • Take as much recovery as you need between sets and exercises • 5min recovery • Body weight – abs circuit: Russian twist; Plank with leg lift (alternate left/right leg lift); Glute bridge • 5 x 20sec. Take 10sec recovery between each exercise	• Intensity is increased with the last two sets of the pyramid requiring you to summon the energy for some more big lifts.

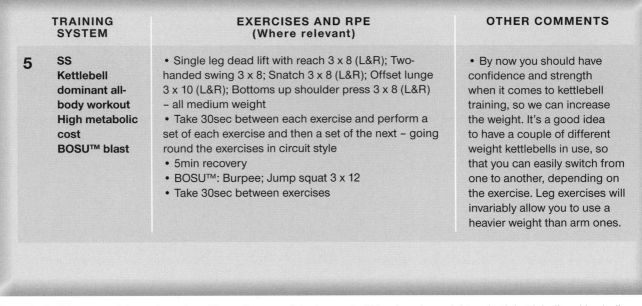

TRAINING SYSTEM	EXERCISES AND RPE (Where relevant)	OTHER COMMENTS
5 **SS** **Kettlebell dominant all-body workout** **High metabolic cost** **BOSU™ blast**	• Single leg dead lift with reach 3 x 8 (L&R); Two-handed swing 3 x 8; Snatch 3 x 8 (L&R); Offset lunge 3 x 10 (L&R); Bottoms up shoulder press 3 x 8 (L&R) – all medium weight • Take 30sec between each exercise and perform a set of each exercise and then a set of the next – going round the exercises in circuit style • 5min recovery • BOSU™: Burpee; Jump squat 3 x 12 • Take 30sec between exercises	• By now you should have confidence and strength when it comes to kettlebell training, so we can increase the weight. It's a good idea to have a couple of different weight kettlebells in use, so that you can easily switch from one to another, depending on the exercise. Leg exercises will invariably allow you to use a heavier weight than arm ones.

Intensity builds across this week again, with another consistent move to lifting heavier weights – both kettlebell and barbell.

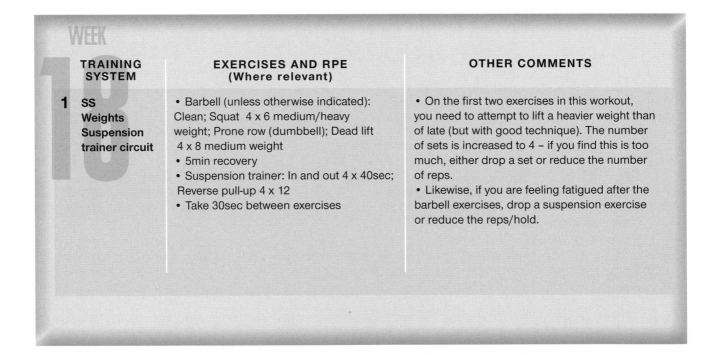

WEEK 13

TRAINING SYSTEM	EXERCISES AND RPE (Where relevant)	OTHER COMMENTS
1 **SS** **Weights** **Suspension trainer circuit**	• Barbell (unless otherwise indicated): Clean; Squat 4 x 6 medium/heavy weight; Prone row (dumbbell); Dead lift 4 x 8 medium weight • 5min recovery • Suspension trainer: In and out 4 x 40sec; Reverse pull-up 4 x 12 • Take 30sec between exercises	• On the first two exercises in this workout, you need to attempt to lift a heavier weight than of late (but with good technique). The number of sets is increased to 4 – if you find this is too much, either drop a set or reduce the number of reps. • Likewise, if you are feeling fatigued after the barbell exercises, drop a suspension exercise or reduce the reps/hold.

	TRAINING SYSTEM	EXERCISES AND RPE (Where relevant)	OTHER COMMENTS
2	**GS Kettlebells Core exercise**	• GS 1: One-handed swing x 10 (L&R); Snatch x 10 (L&R); Single arm clean x 10 (L&R) x 3 • 3min recovery • GS 2: Racked front squat x 20; Clean and press x 10 (L&R); Offset lunge x 10 (L&R) x 3 • Take 45sec between each GS • All with medium weight • 3min recovery • Side plank advanced option 3 x 20sec (L&R)	• Try to increase the weight of the kettlebell/s you use if you can.
3	**CV Sprints**	• 10 x 10sec sprints at RPE 7/8 • 2min walk recovery at RPE 2–4	• Again, you could replace this session with stadium step sprints, taking one or two at a time, if you wanted a change, or do a bike workout as described previously.
4	**P Weights and Body weight abs circuit**	• Barbell (unless otherwise indicated): Sumo squat; Bent over row; Rear foot elevated split squat (dumbbell) • 10 x light weight • 8 x medium weight • 2 x 6 x medium/heavy weight • Take sufficient recovery to be able to complete the lifts • 5min recovery • Body weight – abs circuit: Russian twist; Reverse crunch; Glute bridge 3 x 20sec • Take 10sec recovery between each exercise	• More heavier lifting – the aim of this session is to create optimised conditions for positive hormone production.
5	**SS Kettlebell dominant all-body workout High metabolic cost BOSU™ blast**	• Single leg dead lift with reach 3 x 10 (L&R); Two-handed swing 3 x 10; Snatch 3 x 10 (L&R); Offset lunge 3 x 10 (L&R); Bottoms up shoulder press 3 x 10 • Medium/heavy weight • Take 30sec between exercises and move in circuit style from one to the next • 5min recovery • BOSU™: Bicycle crunch; Jump squat 3 x 12 • Take 30secs between exercises	• With the kettlebells, aim for a fluent, dynamic but controlled workout. A similar session to the one you completed at the end of the previous week.

More of the same structure but there's a progression again this week in terms of intensity – you're lifting more weight!

	TRAINING SYSTEM	EXERCISES AND RPE (Where relevant)	OTHER COMMENTS
1	**SS** **Weights** **Suspension trainer circuit**	• Barbell (unless otherwise indicated): Clean 4 x 10; Dead lift 4 x 10; Bent over row 4 x 10; Squat 4 x 10. Medium weight • Take 1min between exercises and move through set by set. Recover as necessary • Suspension trainer: In and out 4 x 40sec; Reverse pull-up 4 x 12; Chest press 4 x 12; Diagonal reverse crunch 4 x 12 • Take 30sec between exercises	• If your form starts to fail on the barbell exercises, then reduce the weight attempted. This is meant to be a tough session. However, try not to increase the recovery between exercises. • If you are 'feeling it' after the barbell exercises, then reduce the intensity of the suspension part.
2	**GS** **Kettlebells**	• GS 1: One-handed swing x 14 (L&R); Snatch x 14 (L&R); Clean x 14 (L&R) x 3 (Take 45sec at the end of each GS) • 3min recovery • GS 2: Racked front squat x 20; Clean and press x 10 (L&R); Offset lunge x 10 (L&R) x 3 (take 45sec at the end of each GS) • All with light to medium weight • 3min recovery • Side plank advanced option 3 x 20sec (L&R) 30sec recovery between exercises	• Keep the exercises fluent and always brace your core, where relevant. Note: You should use lighter kettlebells today compared to previous similar sessions – this will make for more of a strength endurance workout.
3	**CV** **Sprints**	• 10 x 10sec sprints at RPE 7/8 • 2min walk recovery at RPE 2–4	• Again, you could replace this session with stadium step sprints, taking one or two at a time, or do an exercise bike session if you wanted a change.
4	**SuS** **Weights** **Dynamic barbell/ dumbbell and plyometric combo** **Body weight abs circuit**	• Weights: SuS 1: Barbell clean 4 x 6 and Jump squat 4 x 8 • SuS 2: Barbell sumo squat 4 x 6 and Sumo jump 4 x 8 • SuS 3: Rear foot elevated split squat (dumbbell) 4 x 6 (L&R) and Jump lunge 4 x 10 (L&R) • Use a medium/heavy weight where relevant and take 30sec between each exercise in the superset • Recover as necessary • Body weight – abs circuit: Russian twist; Plank with leg lift (alternate left/right leg lifts); Glute bridge 3 x 30sec – take 10sec recovery between each exercise	• This is a 'complex' super-set. This is a pairing of exercises that combines a jumping exercise with a weights one. The benefits? They target the muscle fibres that will increase lean muscle (fast twitch fibre). And if you are a sports performer, your speed and power will benefit. • You finish up with a body weight circuit.

More positive progression and the addition of a new type of superset (dynamic) just to keep you on your toes!

TRAINING SYSTEM	EXERCISES AND RPE (Where relevant)	OTHER COMMENTS
1 **SS** **Weights** **Suspension trainer circuit**	• Weights: Barbell (unless otherwise indicated): Clean; Dead lift; Bent over row; Squat 4 x 10 • Use a medium weight • Take 1min between exercises and keep moving through them • 5min recovery • Suspension trainer: In and out 4 x 40sec; Reverse pull-up 4 x 12; Chest press 4 x 12; Plank 4 x 30sec hold • Take 30sec between exercises	• Make sure you are fully recovered before you tackle the suspension trainer part of the workout.
2 **GS** **Kettlebells**	• GS 1: One-handed swing x 10 (L&R); Snatch x 10 (L&R); Clean x 10 (L&R) x 4 (take 45sec at the end of each GS) • 3min recovery • GS 2: Racked front squat x 20; Clean and press x 10 (L&R); Offset lunge x 10 (L&R) x 4 (take 45sec at the end of each GS) • All with light/medium weight • 3min recovery • Side plank advanced option 4 x 20sec (L&R) • Take 20sec between sets	• Maintain fluency of exercises – move with the kettlebell, where applicable. The sets have been increased to 4, so it's a progression from last week.
3 **CV** **Sprints**	• 10 x 10sec sprints at RPE 7/8 • 2min walk recovery at RPE 2–4	• If you want a further change, find a hill (tarmac, preferably) with a light grade and perform the workout there.
4 **SS** **Weights** **Suspension trainer**	• Weights: • Barbell clean; Squat; 4 x 4–6 heavy weight • Dumbbell prone row; Dead lift; 4 x 8 medium/heavy weight • 5min recovery • Suspension trainer: In and out 4 x 40sec; Reverse pull-up 4 x 12 • Take 30sec or so between exercises	• Note that the two barbell exercises require a heavy weight to be attempted. If you perform 6 reps on the first set, increase the weight you attempt for the next set, as you will probably have underestimated what you can lift initially.

TRAINING SYSTEM	EXERCISES AND RPE (Where relevant)	OTHER COMMENTS
5 **SuS** **Weights** **Dynamic** **Barbell/** **dumbbell** **and** **plyometric** **combo** **Body weight** **abs circuit**	• SuS 1: Barbell clean 4 x 6 and Jump squat 4 x 8 • SuS 2: Barbell sumo squat 4 x 6 and Sumo jump 4 x 8 • SuS 3: Dumbbell rear foot elevated split squat 4 x 6 (L&R) and Jump lunge 4 x 10 (L&R) • Use a medium to heavy weight (where relevant) • Take 30sec between each exercise in each pair and 90sec between supersets. Use a medium/heavy weight where relevant • 5min recovery • Body weight – abs circuit: Russian twist; Scissors; Glute bridge • 3 x 30sec. Take 10sec recovery between each exercise	• Up your weights if you can. Quality – i.e. speed of movement – is key to getting the most out of the dynamic superset, so take more recovery if you feel yourself tiring.

Over the last 20 weeks, your resistance training proficiency, fitness, functional ability, strength and lean body mass will have come on in leaps and bounds. Take a deep breath and congratulate yourself on your achievements thus far as you now move into the final phase.

Smith machine

A Smith machine is a sturdy frame within which you can perform exercises such as the squat and dead lift, with no need for a training partner ('spotter') on hand to help if you begin to struggle during a lift. With a Smith machine you can halt the lift yourself by rotating the bar so that it hooks on to evenly spaced pegs in its frame – thus preventing the bar from falling.

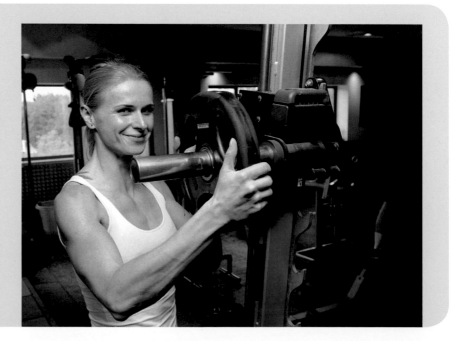

⚖ Weeks 21–24 Resisting - Advanced 3

You are now moving into the final 4 weeks of the 24-week programme. You'll tackle some tough workouts – ones you could only have dreamed about doing when you first embarked on your resistance training journey. A couple of new training systems are also introduced – these are forced reps (FR) and negatives (NR).

They may be two systems you would have steered well clear of before you started resistance training, perhaps because you thought they were way too advanced or even that they were for 'men only' and for body builders at that. They're not! These systems should be seen as further ways to unlock the calorie burning potential of a lean and toned body. They're also great ways to break through a potential training plateau (when you get stuck at a certain weight and your strength seems to have maxed out). However, due to their very intense nature they should only be used sparingly.

WEEK 21	TRAINING SYSTEM	EXERCISES AND RPE (Where relevant)	OTHER COMMENTS
1	**NR Weights SS**	• Weights: Squat; Shoulder press (barbell) 6 x 2 reps with a 5–6sec lower time • Medium/heavy–heavy weight • Take 30sec between each set (of two reps) • 5min recovery • SS: Clean 4 x 5–6 heavy weight • Take as much recovery as you need to complete the lifts – if you begin to fatigue, reduce the number of reps completed	• There are only three exercises in this workout but it's a very intense one. Judge your effort and the weight you use to get through the session of negatives. The weight should be light enough to enable you to be able to push it up yourself.
2	**GS Kettlebells**	• GS 1: One-handed swing x 12 (L&R); Snatch x 12 (L&R); Single-hand clean x 12 (L&R) x 4 (take 45sec at the end of each GS) • 3min recovery • GS 2: Racked front squat x 20; Clean and press x 10 (L&R); Offset lunge x 10 • Take 45sec at the end of each GS • All medium weight • 3min recovery • Side plank advanced option 3 x 20sec (L&R) • Take 20sec recovery between exercises	• Reps are increased from last week. This is a high volume workout.

TRAINING SYSTEM	EXERCISES AND RPE (Where relevant)	OTHER COMMENTS
3 CV Sprints	• 10 x 10sec sprints at RPE 7/8 • 2min walk recovery at RPE 2–4	• As before, you could replace this session with stadium step sprints, taking one or two at a time, an exercise bike workout or hill sprints if you wanted a change.
4 P Weights and SS Body weight abs circuit	• Weights: Barbell (unless otherwise indicated): Sumo squat; Bent over row; Rear foot elevated split squat (dumbbell) • 10 x light weight • 8 x medium weight • 2 x 4 medium/heavy weight • 5min recovery • Body weight – abs circuit: Russian twist; Plank with leg lift; Toe tap • 3 x 30sec • Take 10sec recovery between each exercise	• More weights progression.
5 Weights Dynamic SuS Barbell/ Dumbbell and plyometric combo SS Body weight abs circuit	• SuS 1: Clean 4 x 8 (L&R); Jump squat 4 x 10 • SuS 2: Barbell sumo squat 4 x 6 and Sumo jump 4 x 8 • SuS 3: Dumbbell rear foot elevated split squat 4 x 6 (L&R) and Jump lunge 4 x 10 (L&R) • Use a medium/heavy weight where relevant • Take 30sec between each exercise in each superset and 90sec between supersets • 5min recovery • Body weight – abs circuit: Reverse crunch; Press-up plank; Glute bridge; Scissors • 3 x 30sec • Take 10sec recovery between exercises	• A variation on the dynamic superset theme with a mix of kettlebell, body weight and barbell exercises.

An intense week in terms of the weight lifted and the introduction of some new dynamic superset combinations and negative reps. The mix of sessions is designed to target the muscle fibres that will most respond to creating greater leanness and create a high metabolic cost. Remember that calorie burning lasts long after your workout. And with the progression of training and the level you have reached, your metabolic rate should now be turned on high 24/7.

TRAINING SYSTEM	EXERCISES AND RPE (Where relevant)	OTHER COMMENTS
1 NR SS Barbell	• NR: Barbell front squat and shoulder press 6 x 3 reps with a 6–8sec lower time • Use Medium/heavy–heavy weight • Take 30sec between each set (of three reps) • 5min recovery • SS: Clean 4 x 4; Dead lift 4 x 4 • Heavy weight • Take as much recovery as you need to complete the lifts – if you begin to fatigue, reduce the number of reps completed or pause and start again	• The NRs have been increased and you should attempt to train with a heavier weight compared to last week. • The reps for the Clean and Dead lift have been reduced to 4 (from 5), to allow you the opportunity to really try to lift the heaviest weight you can/have. With around 4 months of resistance training behind you, you'll never have been better placed!
2 GS Kettlebells	• GS 1: One-handed swing x 12 (L&R); Snatch x 12 (L&R); Clean x 12 (L&R) x 4 • Take 45sec at the end of the GS • 3min recovery • GS 2: Racked front squat x 20; Clean and press x 10 (L&R); Offset lunge x 10 (L&R) x 4 • Take 45sec at the end of the GS • 3min recovery • Side plank advanced option 3 x 30sec (L&R) • Take 40sec recovery between exercises • All with medium weight	• The weight you are now able to use will be well in excess of the weight that you used weeks back.
3 CV Sprints	• 10 x 10sec sprints at RPE 7/8 • 2min walk recovery at RPE 2–4	• As before, you could replace this session with stadium step sprints, taking one or two at a time, or do an exercise bike session or hill sprints if you wanted a change.
4 P Weights Body weight abs circuit	• Weights: Barbell (unless otherwise indicated) Front squat; Bent over row; Rear foot elevated split squat (dumbbell) • 8 x light weight • 6 x medium weight • 2 x 4 medium/heavy weight • 2 x 2 very heavy weight • 10 min recovery • Body weight – abs circuit: Russian twist; Scissors; Glute bridge: Press-up plank • 3 x 20sec. Take 10sec recovery between exercises	• A slight tweak to the workout – the last 2 sets of 2 reps are with a very heavy weight. Use a Smith machine/training partner to assist you, where relevant.

TRAINING SYSTEM	EXERCISES AND RPE (Where relevant)	OTHER COMMENTS
5 SuS Dynamic Barbell/ dumbbell and plyometric combo Body weight abs circuit	• Weights: • SuS 1: Kettlebell clean 4 x 8 (L&R) and Jump squat 4 x 10 • SuS 2: Barbell sumo squat 4 x 6 and Sumo jump 4 x 8 • SuS 3: Dumbbell rear foot elevated split squat 4 x 6 (L&R) and Jump lunge 4 x 10 (L&R) • Use a medium/heavy weight where relevant • Take 30sec between each exercise in each superset and 90sec between supersets • 10min recovery • Body weight – abs circuit: Reverse crunch; Press-up plank; Glute bridge; Scissors • 3 x 30sec. Take 10sec recovery between exercises	• The heavy weight and jumping exercises again optimally target your fast twitch muscle fibres.

A slight increase in the intensity of this week's programme, but it's one that you'll be able to handle by now.

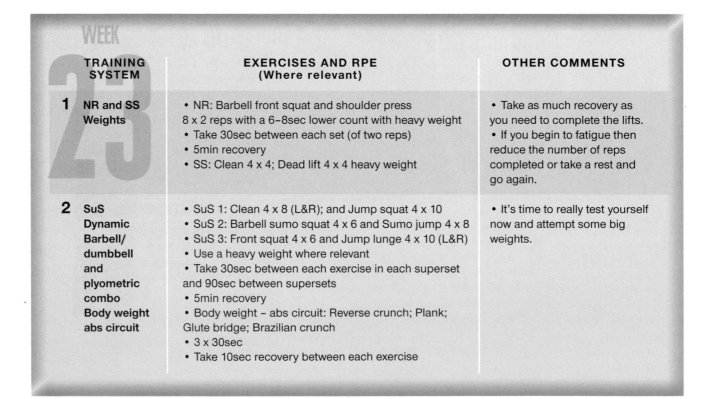

WEEK 23

TRAINING SYSTEM	EXERCISES AND RPE (Where relevant)	OTHER COMMENTS
1 NR and SS Weights	• NR: Barbell front squat and shoulder press 8 x 2 reps with a 6–8sec lower count with heavy weight • Take 30sec between each set (of two reps) • 5min recovery • SS: Clean 4 x 4; Dead lift 4 x 4 heavy weight	• Take as much recovery as you need to complete the lifts. • If you begin to fatigue then reduce the number of reps completed or take a rest and go again.
2 SuS Dynamic Barbell/ dumbbell and plyometric combo Body weight abs circuit	• SuS 1: Clean 4 x 8 (L&R); and Jump squat 4 x 10 • SuS 2: Barbell sumo squat 4 x 6 and Sumo jump 4 x 8 • SuS 3: Front squat 4 x 6 and Jump lunge 4 x 10 (L&R) • Use a heavy weight where relevant • Take 30sec between each exercise in each superset and 90sec between supersets • 5min recovery • Body weight – abs circuit: Reverse crunch; Plank; Glute bridge; Brazilian crunch • 3 x 30sec • Take 10sec recovery between each exercise	• It's time to really test yourself now and attempt some big weights.

TRAINING SYSTEM	EXERCISES AND RPE (Where relevant)	OTHER COMMENTS
3 CV Sprints	• 10 x 15sec sprints at RPE 7–9 • 2min walk recovery at RPE 2–4	• As before, you could replace this session with stadium step sprints, taking one or two at a time, exercise bike sprints or hill sprints, if you wanted a change.
4 P Weights Body weight circuit	• Weights: Barbell (unless otherwise indicated) Front squat; Prone row (dumbbell); Dumbbell rear foot elevated split squat • 8 x light weight • 6 x medium weight • 2 x 4 medium/heavy weight • 2 x 2 very heavy weight • 5min recovery • Body weight circuit: Press-up; Glute bridge; Plank with leg lift (alternate left/right leg lifts); Groiners; 3 x 20sec. Take 10sec recovery between each exercise	• The intensity is upped again.
5 SS Weights Suspension trainer circuit	• Weights: Barbell (unless otherwise indicated) Clean; Dead lift; Barbell bent over row; Squat • 4 x 12 medium weight • Take 1min between exercises and keep moving through them • 5min recovery • Suspension trainer: In and out 3 x 40sec; Reverse pull-up 3 x 12; Chest press 3 x 12 • Take 30sec between exercises	• An increase of 2 reps for the SS will add to the progression from previous similar workouts. • A set of the suspension trainer exercises has been dropped to balance intensity.

You continue to develop your resistance training ability over the penultimate week of the programme, with the emphasis on bigger lifts.

WEEK 24

It's here! Pat yourself on the back (but save the biggest congratulations until the end of the week!) – 24 weeks of resistance training is nearly completed. And it's likely that the progression you have made will be far in excess of what you thought you could achieve. Getting this far should have changed your mind, muscles and body in terms of what you thought was and is possible and it's all down to resistance training – and, of course, you!

	TRAINING SYSTEM	EXERCISES AND RPE (Where relevant)	OTHER COMMENTS
1	P Weights Body weight abs circuit	• Weights: Barbell (unless otherwise indicated) Squat; Prone row (dumbbell); Rear foot elevated split squat (dumbbell) • 6 x medium weight • 2 x 4 medium/heavy weight • 3 x 2 very heavy weight • 5 min recovery • Body weight – abs circuit: Russian twist; Press-up plank; Leg lift; Glute bridge; Reverse crunch • 4 x 20sec. Take 10sec recovery between each exercise	• A continuation from last week's similar workout, although the loading across the pyramid has shifted to more heavier sets (the light/medium first set being dropped and an additional very heavy set of two added). • The abs circuit has also increased in difficulty.
2	SS Weights BOSU™	• Weights: Barbell (unless otherwise indicated) Clean; Dead lift; Bent over row: Front squat; Offset lunge (dumbbell); 4 x 12 (L&R) medium weight • Take 1min between exercises • 5min recovery • BOSU™: Forward lunge 4 x 10 (L&R); Single leg lift with shoulder-press (light weight) 4 x 10 (L&R); BOSU™ squat jump • Take 30sec between exercises	• This is a continuation of the high metabolic cost workouts that you have been following in this phase.
3	CV Sprints	• 10 x 15sec sprints min at RPE 7/8 • 2min walk recovery at RPE 2–4	• You may wonder why the reps have remained at 10 over the workout phases. With this type of training, quality is key and too many reps could eat into this and reduce the power you generate.
4	SS Weights	• Weights: Barbell (unless otherwise indicated) Clean; Dead lift; Squat; Bent over row; Offset lunge (dumbbell); 6 x 12 medium weight • Take 1min between exercises and keep moving through them	• An out and out metabolic and hormonal booster of a session. The additional 2 sets and short recoveries will make for a tough workout – hence there's no second part to this workout.

TRAINING SYSTEM	EXERCISES AND RPE (Where relevant)	OTHER COMMENTS
5 SuS Weights Dynamic Barbell/ dumbbell and plyometric combo Body weight abs circuit	• SuS 1: Kettlebell clean and press 4 x 10 (L&R); Jump squat 4 x 10 • SuS 2: Barbell sumo squat 4 x 8; Sumo jump squat 4 x 8 • SuS 3: Dumbbell rear foot elevated split squat 4 x 8 (L&R); Jump lunge 4 x 10 (L&R) • Use a medium/heavy weight where relevant • Take 30sec between each exercise in each pair and 90sec between supersets • 5min recovery • Body weight – abs circuit: Reverse crunch; Press-up plank; In and out • 3 x 30sec. Take 10sec recovery between exercises	• The body weight circuit has been slightly reduced in intensity to compensate and balance the week's intensity.

You've done it! And you should be very, very proud of yourself. Not only have you completed the 24-week plan, but you will now be very familiar with exercises, training systems and ways of training that were probably quite foreign to you not many weeks ago. Your body will be in great shape and reflecting exactly what resistance training can do.

THE COMPLETE WORK SELFIE

Maybe it's time you changed taking that selfie to a proper photoshoot so you really have a reminder of how far your body has developed over the course of the 24-week training plan. Whatever you decide, you should be looking and feeling great and have a body that you are truly proud of and confident in.

▶ Where to next?

After you have completed the workouts in this book, you could move to a more CV-orientated period of training, (although still containing resistance workouts) for 6–8 weeks. The idea would be to maintain your lean muscle gains while increasing your heart and lung efficiency.

It's very likely that you will, for example, be able to run faster due to the increased strength, power and speed you have developed (remember those near-weekly sprint workouts).

An alternative would be to recommence the programme from weeks 12 through to 24. You could up your weights lifted, where relevant, to ensure continued progression.

Or you could use the knowledge in this book and the experience you have gained over the last 24 weeks to construct your own resistance training workouts (you will find further helpful information in this respect in the next chapter).

It's important that you understand how your body responds and develops to your workouts so you can select the best workout options for you in future – that's why, as I've stressed, that training diary you've been keeping will be so very useful.

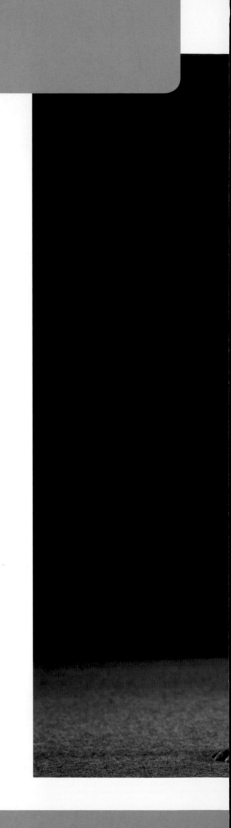

6 MAKE IT A HIT!

⚫ More resistance training ideas

There has been a big change in many people's attitudes in recent years as to how they should train. CrossFit® – with its workouts of the day (aka WODs) and its 'fit for anything' mantra – has done much to make people aware of more intense and, in some cases, extreme methods of training. CrossFit uses High Intensity training (HIT), which relies on quick and powerful movements and exercises, often performed with little or no recovery. In this chapter, we take a look at this type of training and how you can use it and adapt it to benefit your resistance training and take your fitness and body to another level.

The information will provide you with more training options and further knowledge of where and how you can progress your training and what you can incorporate in future.

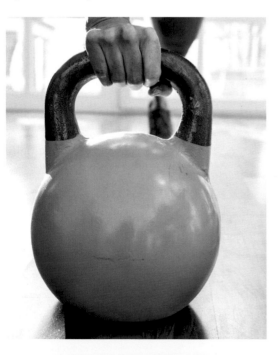

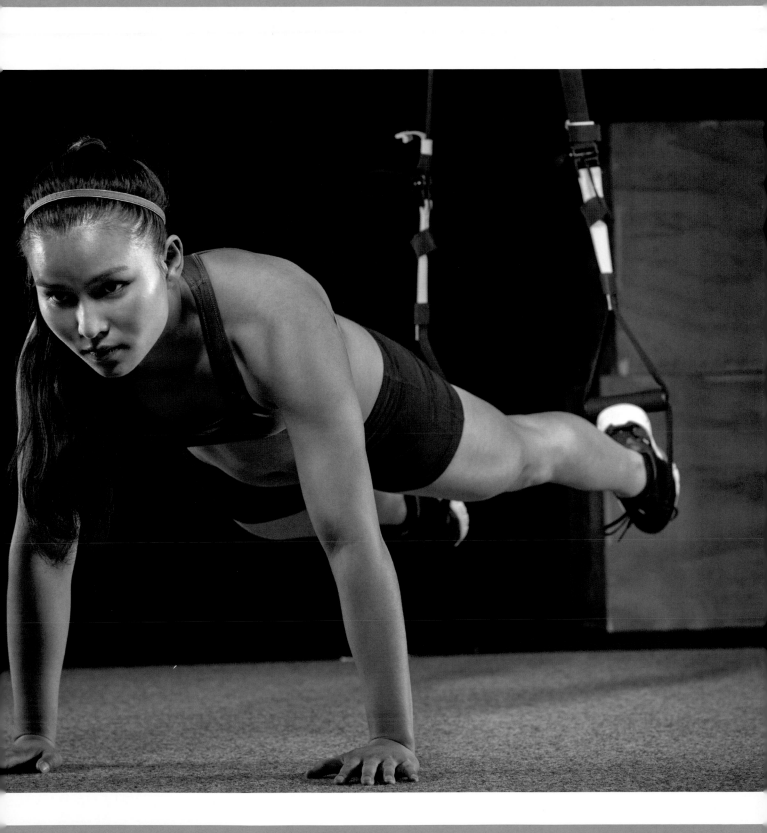

▶ High Intensity Training

HIT (or HIIT – High Intensity Interval Training) has become very popular with personal trainers and in gyms and health clubs, and through CrossFit in recent years, although the concept has been around for a very long time. Circuit training – bursts of high-powered exercises, such as press-ups and burpees, combined with short recoveries – is perhaps the original format of what's become known as HIT. Some of the resistance workouts in this book could easily be labelled HIT workouts, such as the Giant Set kettlebell workouts included in weeks 13–24 of the programme (Chapter 5). Perhaps the key benefits of these types of workouts for weight loss and fat burning and shaping a great body are the elevation they give to metabolic rate through EPOC (see page 15), aka the 'after-burn', and the hormonal stimulation they provide, which can lead to increased lean muscle.

Other benefits of HIT training include increases in strength, power and agility and the fact that they are often quick and easy to do. You could put together a workout from the body weight exercises in Chapter 4 coupled with a training system, such as Circuit Training, escalating Density Training or Giant Sets (see Chapter 3), and do this workout in a park or even your living room! Obviously, the more dynamic the exercises and the more reps and sets and less recovery you take, the more demanding these workouts become.

▶ Plyometric exercises are a great inclusion in a HIT workout due to their dynamic nature, high metabolic cost and do-virtually-anywhere nature.

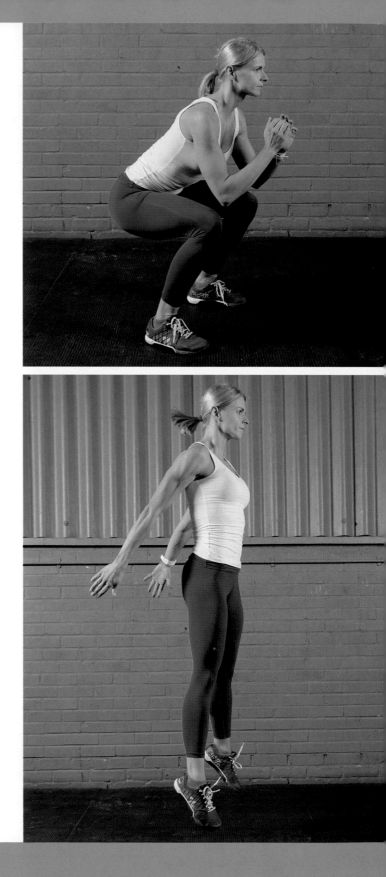

Tabata™ training

Tabata™ training is a specific type of HIT workout, comprising 8 x 20sec flat-out efforts with just a 10-second recovery between each. This very high-intensity form of training was, in the main, the brainchild of Japanese professor Izumi Tabata. Tabata discovered that the HIT method was particularly suited to improving fitness levels – both aerobically and anaerobically – through researching exercise on a stationary bike.

IT'S OVER VERY QUICKLY
... ALTHOUGH IT'S VERY TOUGH

Excluding warm-up and cool-downs, a Tabata™ workout can be completed in just 4 minutes.

The Tabata™ method has garnered improvements of over 28 per cent in fitness even with elite athletes, which is impressive given the difficulty in achieving this with people who are already fit.

Tabata™ training is a very tough workout, but if you have completed the 24 weeks of the programmes in this book you will be in a good position to tackle these workouts. They are great for giving your mind and muscles a real shock (in a positive way!) that could very quickly boost your fitness and are, of course, great time savers – although you may well feel the workout lasted a lot longer than the 230sec it actually took to complete!

Tabata™ workouts should only be performed on a limited basis for everyday fitness trainers and you should approach them with caution as they are very tough.

Some gyms have launched Tabata™ branded classes and these utilise the HIT principle with limited recoveries. You'll get more than 230 seconds worth of effort for your money though!

Here are some examples of Tabata™-style workouts that you could experiment with. For a 'true' Tabata™ workout, you need to work out at an extremely high level of intensity – this means that each 20sec burst should be at near to maximum heart rate. However, it's always best to start at a lower intensity, build confidence and fitness over time, and then 'go for it' when you're ready.

▼ Try sled-pushing for a tough Tabata training work out.

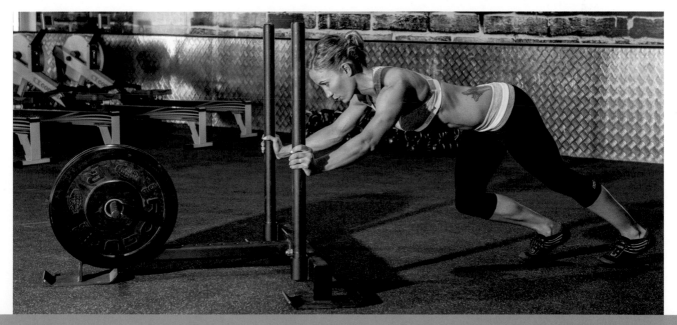

TABATA™-STYLE RESISTANCE WORKOUTS

The most important factor to consider when choosing exercises to use within the Tabata™ training method is to ensure that there is minimal set-up requirement (you only have 10 seconds between sets, remember) and that, technically, you can perform the exercise under stress when severely fatigued. Multi-joint exercises are best as they stress numerous muscles simultaneously and place the greatest demand on your cardiovascular system. You'll find many suitable exercise options within the exercises used in this book (see Chapters 4 and 5). In terms of added resistance exercises, the kettlebell clean and press and snatches are highly applicable – but you must be able to hold form (you could have a variety of weight kettlebells to use for the 8 intervals, reducing the weight you use as you fatigue, for example). Expect to feel sore for a few days after a Tabata™-style workout and make sure you cool down thoroughly and have an easier session or a rest day the day after.

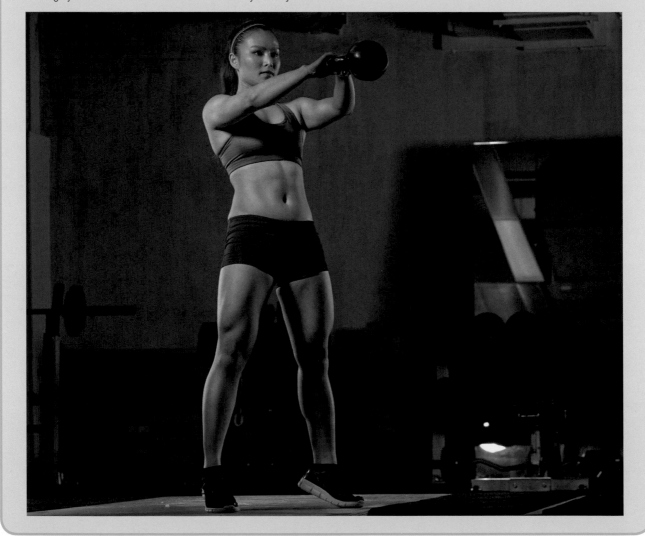

CrossFit®

CrossFit® is the brainchild of Greg Glassman, a gymnastics coach based in California who set up his gym in Santa Cruz over 20 years ago. After studying the training routines of many elite athletes, he realised that compound exercises coupled with high-intensity movement are key to great fitness. He accordingly developed CrossFit®, which meshes together these elements of fitness and his 'philosophy' to produce one of the biggest fitness phenomena of all-time. CrossFit® includes power lifting, Olympic weightlifting, gymnastics, running and kettlebell training, for example. Many have questioned the safety of CrossFit® principles; however, sponsored national and international CrossFit® Games and 5,500 affiliate gyms (or 'boxes', as they are called) worldwide prove the appeal of the 'fit for and ready for anything' approach of CrossFit®.

With the strength, power and agility you will have achieved after completing the 24-week resistance training programme in this book, you will be ideally placed to do a bit of CrossFit® or even take it up seriously, join a box and enter CrossFit® competitions.

▼ Below: a CrossFit style gym, or box.

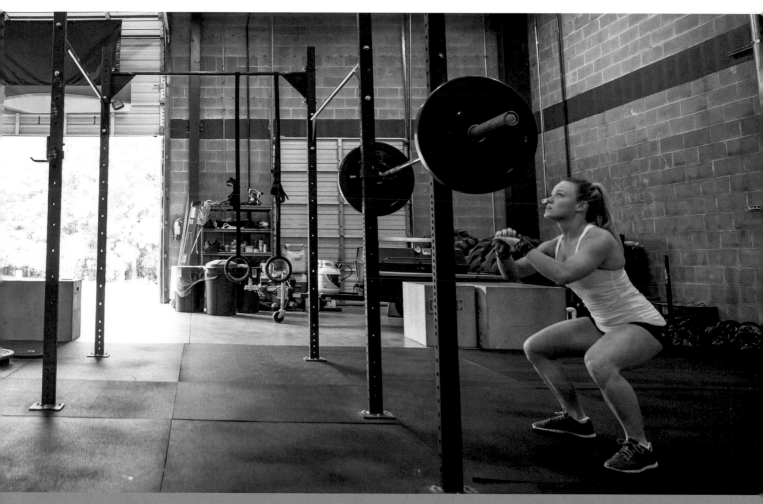

Christine Cope

36-YEAR OLD MOTHER OF TWO AND
CROSSFIT® ADVOCATE

'I'd seen loads of stuff on the internet about CrossFit® and thought it looked cool but was way out of my reach. Even though I knew there was a gym on my doorstep, it took six months before I built up the courage to get in touch. Now it's like my second home. It's an amazing community, more like a club than a gym.

'At first the workouts and training seemed so difficult but because it's technically challenging it gives me the opportunity to step out of my everyday life and really focus on something I'm doing for me. Before CrossFit® I couldn't do things like lift my children over my head and put them on my shoulders. They're six and eight now and I can lift them no problem. It's also helped me in many practical other ways. If I get a puncture on my car, I'm now strong enough to take the wheel off myself and put the spare on. CrossFit® is very relevant to my everyday life.'

CROSSFIT®-INSPIRED WORKOUT 1

Here's a HIT CrossFit®-inspired workout for you to try. It contains some advanced moves, so please spend time mastering these before going for the complete workout. Indeed, learning some of the exercises will itself be an accomplishment!

If you have a high level of relevant fitness, move straight from one exercise to the next; however, if you fatigue unduly or are at a lower level of specific fitness, take a longer recovery. It's crucial that you perform the exercises safely and with control. The fitter you get, the more circuits you can complete and the less recovery you can take. ▶

CROSSFIT®-INSPIRED WORKOUT 1

Handstand press-up

- Kick yourself up against a wall into a handstand. Keep your body as straight as possible.
- Slowly lower yourself to the floor until your head nearly touches it. Inhale as you do so.
- Push yourself back up as you exhale until your elbows are nearly locked.
- Repeat.

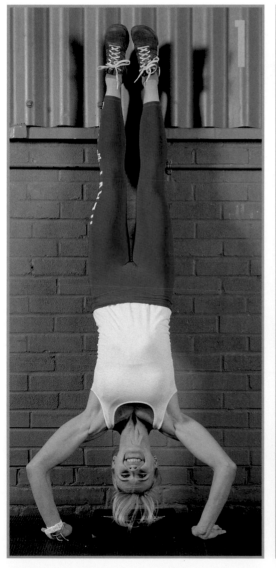

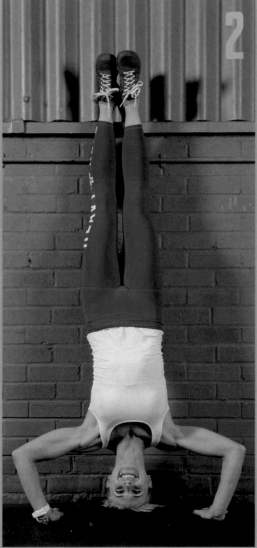

TARGET MUSCLES AND FUNCTIONAL BENEFITS

- Shoulders
- Core strength
- Balance
- Body awareness

3 × 3–5

⊢TIP

Have a training partner/ spotter help you, especially if doing this exercise for the first time. It's of utmost importance that you lower slowly.

TARGET MUSCLES AND FUNCTIONAL BENEFITS

- Rear shoulders
- Upper back
- Latissimus dorsi
- Grip strength

$3 \times 3-5$

Pull ups

- Grab the bar with an over-grasp grip (your palms should face forward).
- With both arms extended and keeping your head facing forward with chin up, slowly pull yourself up until your chin is above the bar.
- Slowly lower yourself back to the starting position (full arms extension).

⫯TIP

Focus on the 'pull' coming from the lats. You can also do negative reps. Have a training partner lift you into the top position or use a box/jump up to grab the bar. Then lower very slowly to the 'arms extended' position. Reset and repeat. This eccentric muscle training will benefit your overall strength.

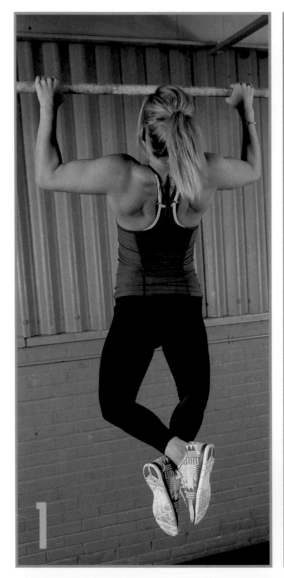

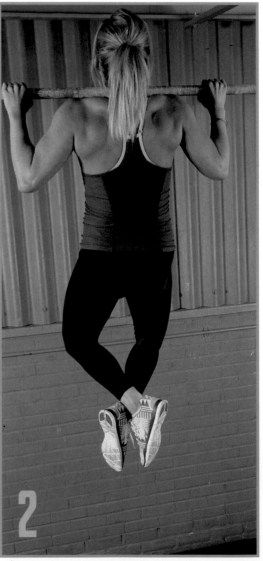

Wall ball

- Stand about 1 metre/3 feet away from a wall with your feet shoulder-width apart. Hold the medicine ball in front of your chest with your arms bent (use a 3–5kg/6½–11lb ball).
- Bend your legs and lower until your thighs are just parallel to the floor – as if performing a squat.
- Explosively extend your arms and legs, bringing your body to a standing position while throwing the ball at your target.
- Gather the ball and repeat.

3 × 10

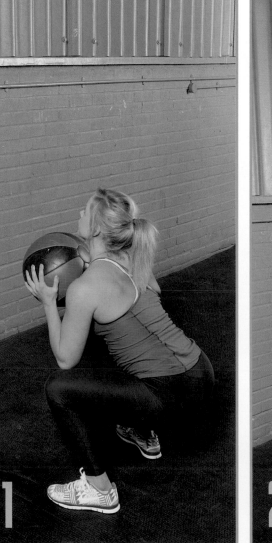

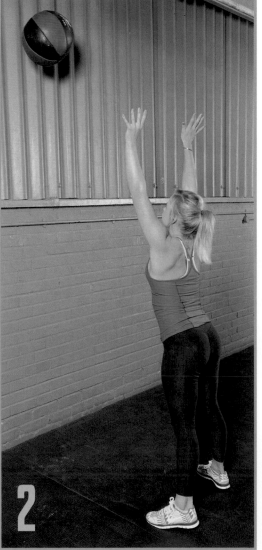

This is a great exercise to boost all-body power and it also has a high metabolic cost.

3 X 1–3
climbs

Rope climbs

■ Wrap the end of the rope under your right foot and around the top of your left foot. This creates a step to begin the climb.

■ Place your left hand on the rope about 15cm/6 inches above the top of your head and grip.

■ Push down with your right foot as you grab the rope with your other hand and lift your left foot off the floor. Both feet are now suspended and your left hand should be holding the rope just above your right hand.

■ Pull yourself up srraight and place your right hand a little higher than the left.

■ Grip the rope between your feet and use your arms to pull yourself up the rope.

■ Repeat these steps until you reach the top with your hands.

■ Reverse your feet and hand positions to climb down slowly.

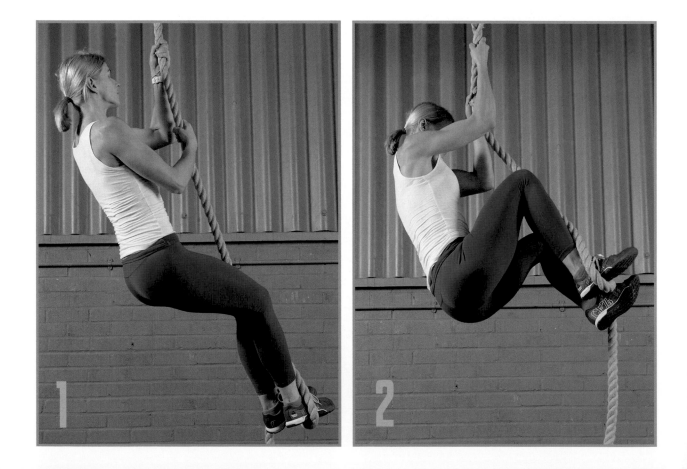

Sled pull

- Load the sled with the desired weight.
- Get into an athletic posture with weight forwards on the balls of your feet and leaning away from the sled with your arms in a running position.
- Pull the sled as fast as possible by driving your legs and arms forwards and backwards. Focus on pulling from your hips.

TARGET MUSCLES AND FUNCTIONAL BENEFITS

- Back
- Glutes
- Hamstrings
- Quads
- Calves

3 x 20m

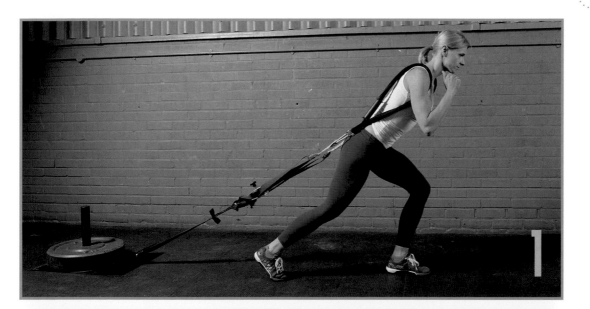

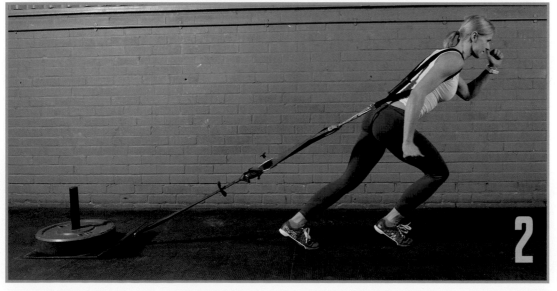

3 × 5 flips

Tyre flips

- Squat behind the tyre, take hold of the rim and, keeping your arms long, drive your legs up to lift the tyre.
- Lean into the movement as the tyre moves to upright and then fully extend your body to drive it up and over, using your arms to add power as you do so.
- Move around the tyre and flip it back the other way as just described.

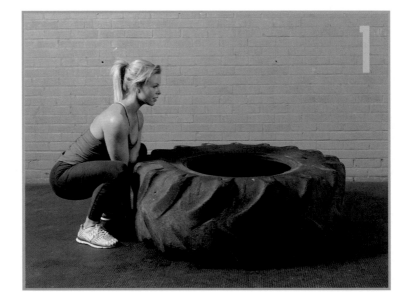

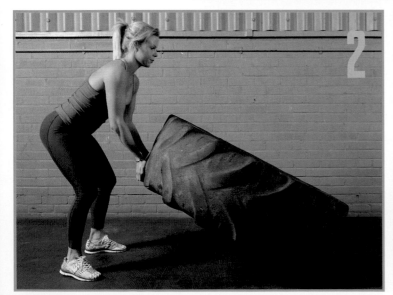

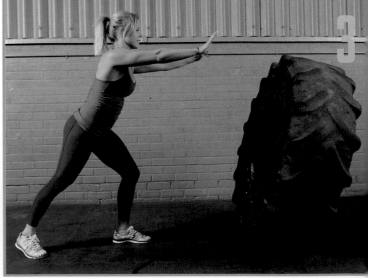

CROSSFIT®-INSPIRED WORKOUT 2

This workout will test various aspects of fitness, strength, power, endurance and your mental toughness. Only attempt this workout if you are relevantly conditioned.

- 500m rowing machine
- 50 step-ups – holding 10kg (22lb) dumbbells
- 20 crunches
- 10 jump squats
- 750m rowing machine
- 50 step-ups – holding 10kg (22lb) dumbbells
- 20 crunches
- 10 jump squats
- 1,000m rowing machine
- 50 step ups – holding 10kg (22lb) dumbbells
- 20 crunches
- 10 jump squats
- 800m run (can be replaced with row again, treadmill can be used)

To find out more about CrossFit®
go to: www.crossfit.com and
for the CrossFit® games:
http://games.crossfit.com

SPRINT TO BEAT FAT

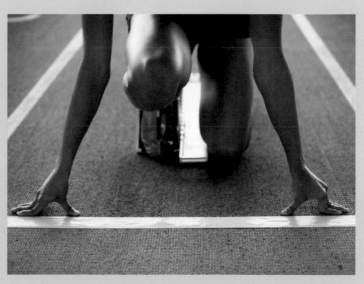

Sprinting is an equally functional exercise and one that I believe is great for developing a great-looking body, too. It's prominent in the 24-week training programme, particularly Chapter 5, as you'll now know! Sprinting uses virtually every muscle in your body and you need to dynamically overcome three times plus your body weight on every stride, so it's a great resistance exercise. Your core is also vitally important for sprinting as it acts to stabilise and transfer the power generated by your legs and arms as you sprint onto the running surface.

As I indicated previously in the practical chapters, if you haven't sprinted for a while you should build up to running flat out and perhaps visit your local athletics club to get some technique and warm up tips in first.

Functional fitness

Functional training, similar to HIT and CrossFit, is also much in vogue. Functional training refers to movements, exercises and exercise systems that reflect real, everyday-life physical (and sports) requirements – not those 'manufactured' in gyms using, for example, fixed path weights machines. Functional training makes your body the machine and your training must optimise its performance for a multitude of movements, strength and endurance tasks. In everyday life we need to stand, reach and turn, bend down and move sideways, reach up and grab an object. These are the movements that functional exercise trains – the movements used when lifting something from the boot of your car, getting up from the floor, digging the garden or carrying a child.

Functional training is obviously key to CrossFit, although the way you train for it does not have to be so intense. The majority of the exercises in the 24-week programme (see Chapters 4 and 5) are also functional in that they integrate your limbs into full body movements and often require skill to complete them. They work your body as it was designed to be.

Functional Fitness-based Workout Programme

TABLE 7

DAY	WORKOUT	COMMENT
Monday	CrossFit™-style workout	Select various exercises that test all elements of fitness. CrossFit-style workout 2 would make for a suitable workout here. Adjust exercise selection and duration to suit your current fitness levels.
Tuesday	Rest	
Wednesday	Tabata™-style workout	Select exercises that you know you will be able to complete for those 8 x 20sec flat-out bursts, with only 10 sec recovery.
Thursday	Rest	
Friday	Sprints	8 x 60m with a full recovery between each, then 10min and finish then a 30m run at 75% effort.
Saturday	CrossFit-style workout	Reduce the intensity slightly compared to the Monday workout. CrossFit-style workout 1 would make a good base for this type of workout. It's more strength-orientated and slightly less taxing, especially if you factor in more recovery.
Sunday	Kettlebell workout	Why not do a giant set kettlebell workout as found in Chapter 5's workout programme? It'll add a further strength and strength endurance element to the programme.

In Table 7 you'll find a week's CrossFit-inspired, HIT and functional-fitness-based workout programme. You could follow/adapt this type of workout progression after you have completed the 24-week programme. By now, with the knowledge and experience you've gained from this book, you should be able to construct highly relevant and targeted workouts for yourself that you'll want to do and, crucially, understand why you are doing them.

Sports training

The benefits of resistance training are integral to sports training and many top-level sportswomen use a myriad of resistance exercises as part of their training programme. Indeed, many of the exercises you will have performed in the practical training chapters of this book are actually sports conditioning exercises (e.g. weights exercises such as the clean, dead lift and squat variations, and plyometric exercises such as the jumping lunge and jump squat). Many of the workouts in Chapters 4 and 5 could easily be used to boost your netball, running and football performance, with little or no adaptation. The key to a sport-specific training programme is really down to the way the workouts are combined with other sports training requirements and how these all fit together in the overall training programme. There's little point, for example, in performing lots of squats if the strength you gain isn't directly transferred into improving your sports performance, so there's no benefit of 'strength for the sake of strength'.

In the next section are some sport-specific relevant exercises. I have included these to show you how resistance training exercises can be adapted to improve sports performance.

If you require a detailed overview of sport-specific training, try these two books: *The Complete Guide to Sports Training* and *Strength Training for Runners*, both published by Bloomsbury.

Sample sports-specific exercises

The two exercises provided can be described as 'evolved' exercises that have been designed very specifically for sports conditioning purposes – however, they could still be used for everyday fitness purposes. Many sports resistance exercises are developed from standard exercises with coach and athlete working out how to make the movement more specific to the needs of their specific sport. This makes what you do in the gym all the more likely to get results when you do your sport.

Box jump with band pull-apart

- Stand with your feet shoulder-width apart, with the band extended and tensioned across your chest.
- Bend your legs and leap up onto the box top, pulling the band apart as you do so while keeping it in broadly the same horizontal position.
- Land, step back down to the floor and repeat.

SPORTS USE Coordinating strong upper body movement with a lower body one is key to a multitude of sports and this exercise does just this.

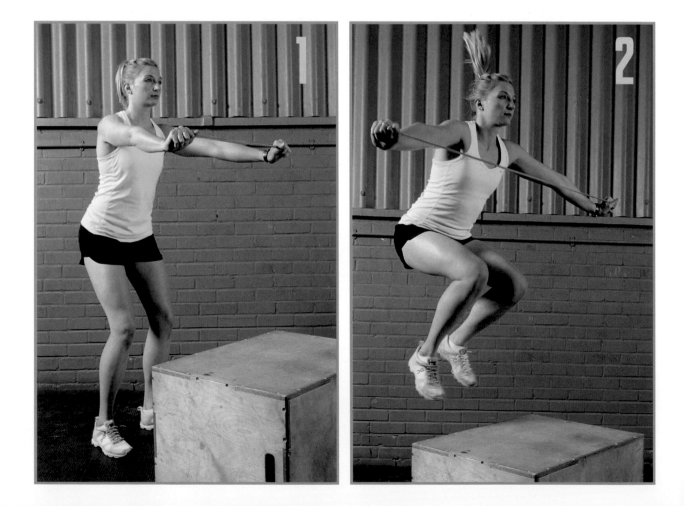

Rotational in-place jumps

- Stand with your feet shoulder-width apart and knees lightly bent.
- Leap up into the air and rotate your hips to the right and then back to straight, keeping your head and shoulders relatively front on as you do so.
- Land and repeat the exercise, twisting to the left.

SPORTS USE Agility is a key aspect of numerous sports and even running requires rotational control and stability. Being able to absorb and react to rotational forces and change of direction is therefore crucial for optimum sports performance.

TARGET MUSCLES AND FUNCTIONAL BENEFITS

- Legs
- Ankles
- Body awareness
- Agility

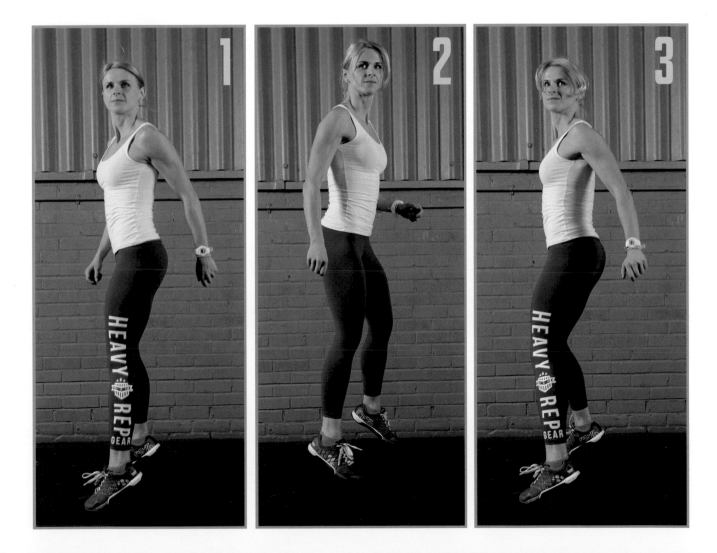

7 RESISTANCE NUTRITION

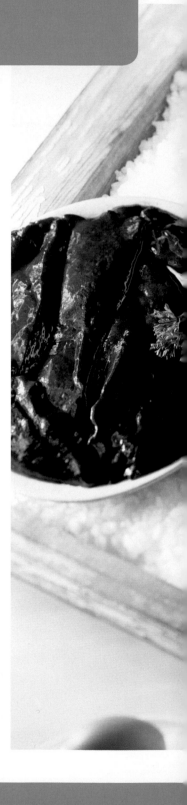

Now you know how to use resistance exercise to shape the body you aspire to (and how to functionally train and potentially devise other training plans), it's time to consider how you fuel it for optimum results. It's been said many times but the truth is that no matter how much training you do, you can't out-train a bad diet.

In this chapter, you'll find out how to calculate your calorie needs and what the key nutrients (macro and micro) are when it comes to sustaining your resistance-training-based fitness lifestyle and why a diet skewed more towards protein than carbs is the best one to support your resistance training, body shaping and metabolic needs. You'll also understand the value of micronutrients (vitamins and minerals) in assisting your training and discover whether it's worth using supplements.

DIETARY TIP

Keep a food diary – it'll provide you with a great starting point for making dietary changes. Be honest and write down everything you eat over a week. This will help you see what you are eating, how much saturated fat you are consuming and whether you're going for low or high energy releasing foods and what your daily calorific consumption is in terms of macronutrients, for example. And, crucially, whether your diet is boosting your training, in terms of recovery and adaptation.

ENERGY RELEASE FROM DIFFERENT FOOD TYPES			
	Carbohydrate	Protein	Fat
Macronutrient /energy in Kcal/g	4	4	9

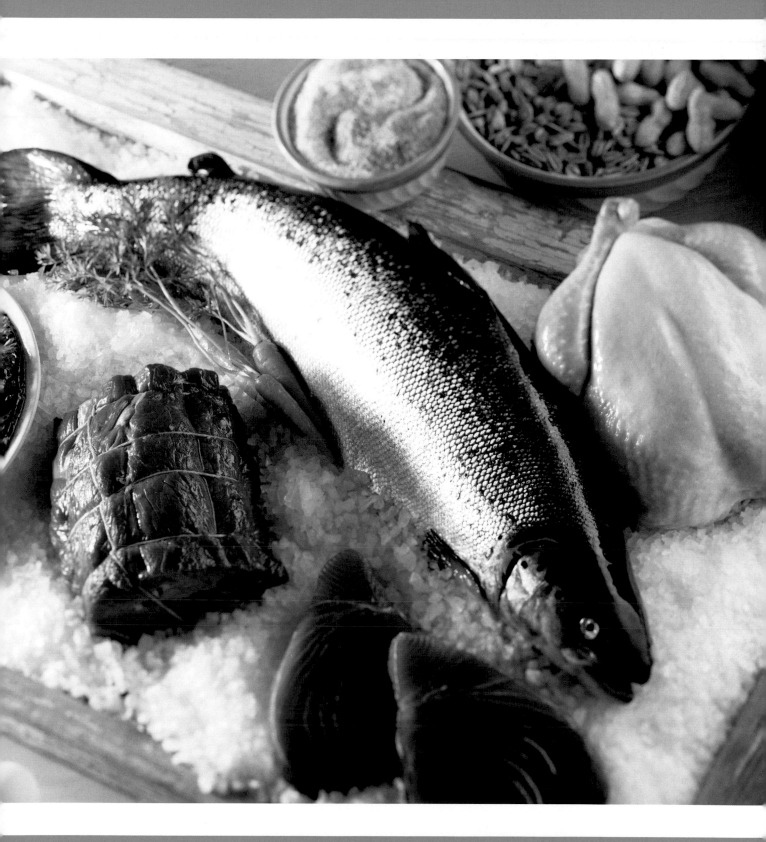

What is a calorie?

Pick up a food product, look at the nutritional information on the label and you'll invariably see that the energy value is expressed in kJ (kilojoules) or j (joules) and/or kcal (kilocalories) or cal (calories).

Understanding food energy

CALORIES

Metric: 1 kcal = 1,000 calories

Imperial: 1 [large] calorie = 1,000 [small] calories

A kcal and a [large] calorie supply the same amount of energy (that's why the terms can be used interchangeably).

One [small] calorie is the amount of heat required to increase the temperature of 1 gram (g) of water by 1 degree centigrade. It's a very small amount of energy, hence the general use of the bigger kcal/calorie unit (a 'calorie' is understood to be a large calorie).

KILOJOULES

The kilojoule is the international standard for energy.
1 kJ = 1,000 joules

A kJ is not the same as a kcal (or calorie) in terms of its energy provision. To facilitate your dietary calculations and ease your understanding of food labels, you can convert kJ into kcal and vice versa by using this calculation:

To convert kJ into kcal, divide by 4.2 – thus 200 kJ = 48 kcal (200/4.2)

To convert kcal into kJ, multiply by 4.2 – thus 100 kcal = 420 kJ (100 x 4.2)

The energy balance equation

Burning fat and losing weight is theoretically very simple – all you need to do is burn more calories than you consume, through diet and/or exercise. If you do this, you'll achieve what's known as a 'positive energy balance' (see Table 8). However, the reality is a little more complex, especially when following a diet designed specifically to benefit your resistance training and develop and maintain the calorie burning potential of lean muscle.

Note: There may be times when you need a negative energy balance (i.e. consume more calories than meets your total energy needs), for example if you are looking to gain weight.

Protein power

Of the three macronutrients (carbs, protein and fat), protein may well be the key macronutrient when it comes to shaping the body you desire and optimising your resistance training and metabolic rate. This is because protein builds and maintains muscles and has a higher thermic effect – that is, your body uses up more energy to metabolise protein compared to fats and carbohydrate.

Note: all the macronutrients produce energy, although carbs are the preferred source for activity.

I previously indicated how too much aerobic training could create a slimmer body, but one that's possibly not toned, strong or functionally fit. The typical macronutrient emphasis for someone who trains this way would be carb-dominant. Indeed, carbs are needed to restock the glycogen (stored muscle carb-fuel) that will be depleted through such training – but in doing so, protein may be overlooked as an important dietary ingredient, and carbohydrate needs may be overestimated.

You'll probably have heard of the Paleo diet – the diet

THE ENERGY BALANCE EQUATION   TABLE 8

Kcal intake	Kcal output	Effect on	Energy balance*
1,600	1,600	None	Balanced
2,000	1,600	Increase	Negative (+400)
1,600	1,900	Decrease	Positive (-300)

*Refers to the difference between calories in and out

PROTEIN AND WEIGHT LOSS

Research indicates that protein (and dairy produce) is important for losing and maintaining weight in obese, active and resistance training women.[12, 13, 14] This is again due to the role played by protein in maintaining and building lean mass (muscle) – mass that has a greater metabolic benefit, burning calories all day and every day.

our prehistoric forebears followed out of necessity. There were no processed, high sugar, salt and fat options and food was in its most organic state (when it could be caught, in terms of animals, or foraged, in terms of plants). Today, the Paleo diet can be described as consisting of foods that would once have been hunted, fished and gathered in woods and forests, such as grass-fed raised meats, fish, vegetables and certain fruits and nuts. A high percentage of meat is one of the key features of the diet. A strict Paleo diet excludes foods that are today farmed and manufactured, such as grains, dairy products and even potatoes. Advocates of the Paleo diet believe that our bodies have not significantly adapted to the higher carbs found in grains, not to mention the chemicals and processing involved in the production of modern foods, and therefore we still work best on a Paleo diet. I'm not going to recommend that you try to stick rigidly to this diet, as it can recommend that 55–65 per cent of daily calories should come from animal foods, and 35–45 per cent from plant foods. However, I am going to suggest that for strength and resistence training you skew your diet in a more general Paleo way, particularly in favour of protein.

Train like an athlete

Although you may not see yourself as an athlete, you should view yourself as one as you complete the 24-week training programme. You will be training progressively intensely, utilising many of the exercises and training systems that athletes do.

Here's some research that backs up the need to consume optimum amounts of protein in your diet to maintain and build lean muscle and lose weight – it focuses on athletes but, given what I've just said, do take note of the recommendations. Researchers looked at how protein could aid weight loss. Initially, they pointed to a large body of evidence indicating that athletes should eat 2–3 times the recommended dietary allowance (RDA) of protein. Their recommendation was 1.8–2.7g per kg (approx. ½–1oz per 2lb) of body weight (0.8g per kg/¼oz per 2lb of body weight is typical for people who don't work out). Equally important was *when* protein was eaten and the researchers suggested that this should be evenly spaced throughout the day. They also suggested that protein should be consumed immediately after a workout to fuel your muscles.[15]

Do you need to protein-supplement?

You can usually get your protein needs from your normal diet, as long as you build in optimum amounts. Lean cuts of meat, fish and dairy will provide you with the majority of what you need. However, as indicated, certain types of protein offer quicker digestive benefits than others and this is where specific supplements can be useful. They're also beneficial from the perspective of ease of use.

For example, protein from whey, a by-product of milk from which many supplements are derived, is more quickly absorbed and therefore more suitable for post-

workout recovery, while casein (the main protein present in milk) is more slowly digested and is more suited to pre-bedtime (your muscles recover and rebuild when you are sleeping, so being 'dripped' protein overnight can aid this process).

PROTEIN RATING (BIOAVILABILITY)

Proteins are given a 'bioavailability' rating, marked out of 100, that indicates their level of inclusion of all the essential amino acids (see opposite). For example, eggs have a protein rating of 100, fish of 70, milk 67 and brown rice 57. Relatively low bioavailability would be indicated by a score under 70.

Turkey, cottage cheese, egg whites, soya beans, semi-skimmed milk and pulses are great low-fat sources of protein. Plant foods are also sources of protein. The following selected options will provide you with around 10g (½oz) of protein:

- 4 slices of wholemeal bread
- 400g (14oz) cooked rice
- 300g (10oz) cooked pasta
- 120g (4oz) tofu
- 60g (2oz) nuts
- 30g (1oz) reduced-fat cheese
- 70g (2½oz) cottage cheese
- 250ml (8 US fl oz) low-fat milk
- 40g (1½oz) lean cooked chicken
- 50g (1¾oz) grilled fish
- 200g (7oz) reduced-fat yogurt

ESSENTIAL AND NON-ESSENTIAL AMINO ACIDS

Essential amino acids	Non-essential amino acids
Isoleucine	Alanine
Leucine	Arginine
Lysine	Asparagine
Methionine	Aspartic acid
Phenylalanine	Cysteine
Threonine	Glutamic acid
Tryptophan	Glutamine
Valine	Glycine
	Histidine (essential for babies only)
	Proline
	Serine
	Tyrosine

Source: Adapted
from Anita Bean's
*The Complete Guide
to Sports Nutrition*
(6th edition).

TABLE 9

Protein can supply energy – albeit in limited amounts

During endurance activities lasting more than an hour,
specific amino acids (valine, leucine and isoleucine) in
muscles are used as a fuel source, as glycogen stores
deplete. At this time, protein can supply 15 per cent of the
body's energy requirements, compared to its normal 5 per
cent when glycogen stores are full.

The ideal post-workout cocktail

Post workout, it's very important that you immediately
kick-start your recovery. Muscles will have been depleted
of glycogen and resistance training will have broken down
muscle protein. Carbohydrate combined with protein is
the ideal post-workout cocktail – one that also creates
the optimal hormonal response of growth hormone and
insulin (see Chapter 3). Insulin is responsible for pushing

amino acids and glucose (sugary carbs) into your muscles.
1:4 = the ideal protein to carbohydrate ratio for your
post-workout snack.

Examples:
- Glass of chocolate milk
- 1–2 portions of fruit and a glass of milk
- 1–2 yogurts
- Jacket potato with tuna, baked beans or cottage cheese
- Fruit and yogurt smoothie

Note: Your body needs all the essential amino acids to
build and maintain muscle. Note also that you would need
to consider the calorific value of your post-workout recovery
meal/drink in terms of your overall calorie consumption.

How much protein do you need?

Most diets actually contain sufficient quantities of protein – and yours should too (if not already) after you have read this chapter and have more fully understood the power of protein.

Serious resistance training (as you will be doing) requires more protein than endurance training – the usual amount required appears to be within the range of 1.6–1.9g (approx. ½oz) of protein per day per kg (2lb) of body weight. However, very recently higher levels are being considered (see 'Train like an athlete', page 192). It's certainly worth considering upping your protein consumption in the second half of the training programme.

So if you weighed 70kg (154lb), you would need to consume between 112g and 133g (4–5oz) of protein per day.

(see 'Train like an athlete', page 192)

TABLE 10

REQUIRED FOOD CONSUMPTION, INCLUDING PROTEIN CONTENT, FOR 70KG (154LB) RESISTANCE TRAINING PERSON

	Quantity of food required to provide needs for a 70 kg athlete	Amount of protein g
Breakfast	300ml milk	12
	2 slices of toast	8
	2 tablespoons jam	0
	250ml juice	2
Lunch	2 bread rolls each with chicken and salad	41
	1 banana	2
	1 fruit bun	6
	250ml flavoured low-fat milk	13
Dinner	Stir-fry with 250g pasta and 100g meat and 250g vegetables	50
	250g jelly and custard	13
Snacks	750ml sports drink	0
	1 carton yogurt	10
	1 piece of fruit	1
	1 cereal bar	2
	Total	160g/6oz (2.3g/kg or 1oz/2lb body weight)

Source: Adapted from www.ausport.gov.au/ais/nutrition/factsheets/basics/protein_–_how_much

Carbohydrate

Carbohydrate is the body's prime fuel source when we are physically active. On digestion, it increases blood sugar levels and provides energy – as we'll see later, some sources of carbohydrate do this more quickly than others. Carbohydrate is also stored in the muscles and liver as glycogen (glycogen, as noted, can be seen as 'premium grade' muscle fuel). The body can only store it in limited amounts – about 375g. It needs to be constantly replenished for us to remain in optimum workout condition and to gain the most from resistance training.

Carbohydrate energy is released through a series of chemical reactions that use glycogen, glucose and oxygen as the starting materials.

SIMPLE AND COMPLEX CARBOHYDRATES

Carbohydrates can be divided into two types – simple (sugars) and complex (fibres and starches). Simple carbohydrates contain one or two sugar units in their molecules, while complex carbohydrates contain from 10 to thousands of sugar units. Many foods contain a mixture of both simple and complex carbohydrates, so to measure their immediate energy release, foods are given a Glycaemic Index (GI) rating. This ranges from 1–100.

Low GI foods release their energy more slowly than high GI foods.

Optimise your energy levels

Knowing the GI of foods can help you to optimise your energy levels throughout the day. If you need a quick boost, then a high GI food is a good choice, while low GI foods eaten regularly throughout the day will provide a steady supply of energy and reduce 'sugar cravings'. The right balance of carbs will therefore keep your metabolism revving nicely.

VEGETARIAN?

If you're a vegetarian, you may not get all the amino acids you need – or at least not so simply. There's little research to indicate that a properly planned and consumed vegetarian diet will hamper fitness or sports performance, but you should aim to eat protein-rich foods that contain all the essential amino acids.

Quinoa is one such food that contains all essential amino acids and a good supply of B vitamins, vitamin E and dietary fibre. It also has a low GI.

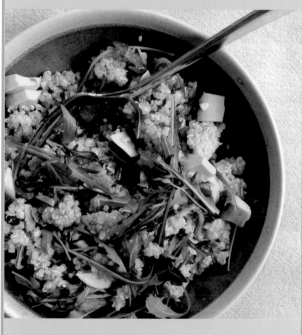

▲ Quinoa is high in protein and low in fat

Three main meals a day and two or three snacks will optimally support your metabolism, your resistance training and any body shaping needs you have.

THE GLYCEAMIC INDEX OF SELECTED CARBOHYDRATES

TABLE 11

Sugars		Fruit and vegetables		Pulses	
Glucose	100	Pineapple	66	Red kidney beans	27
Sucrose	65	Raisins	66	Butter beans	31
		Watermelon	72	Soya beans	18
Bread, rice and pasta		Banana	55		
Bread, white	70	Orange	44		
Bread, wholemeal	69	Plum	39	**Other**	
Pizza	60	Grapes	46	Shortbread	64
Rice, brown	76	Apples	38	Oatmeal	55
Rice, white	87			Ryvita	69
Basmati	58	Baked potato	85	Rice cakes	85
Macaroni	45	Chips	75	Tortillas	72
Instant noodles	46	Boiled potato	56	Muesli bar	61
		Peas	48	Mars bar	68
Breakfast cereals		Carrots	49	Muffin	44
Cornflakes	84	Broad beans	79	Peanuts	14
Weetabix	69				
Muesli	56	**Dairy products**			
Porridge with water	42	Full-fat milk	27		
All-Bran	42	Skimmed milk	32		

Despite its usefulness, GI does have limitations. For a start, it measures the energy release from single foods rather than meals that usually combine different carbohydrates, fats and proteins. This 'mix' can obviously affect energy release.

GI CLASSIFICATION

HIGH GI: Carbs with a GI of 71–100

MEDIUM GI: Carbs with a GI of 56–70

LOW GI: Carbs with a GI of 0–55

▶ Factors to take into account when estimating the energy release of meals in terms of GI

■ Protein and fat reduce GI.

■ For meals that combine two different GI-rated foods in roughly the same quantity, for example, rice and kidney beans, total the GI of the two foods and divide by two. Example: rice GI = 87, kidney beans GI = 27, total GI = 114. Therefore the meal's average GI = 57 (114 divided by 2).

■ The smaller the size of the food particles, the more speedily food is digested and the quicker it will release its energy – hence the high GI of foods such as bread and breakfast cereals. Refined carbs also tend to have a higher GI and are much less wholesome.

Carb requirements to support resistance training

As I've pointed out, protein may be the key macronutrient when it comes to optimising your resistance training. However, if you don't consume the right amount and types of carbs you will also hinder the results of your training. The 24-week workout programme will deplete your muscles' glycogen stores – hence it's important that you consume sufficient carbs throughout the day and equally importantly pre- and post- workout in order to fuel and refuel your body. Do this and you'll have enough energy for your workouts and for your everyday activities. Also, if you allow your blood sugar levels to fluctuate throughout the day your body will be more likely to increase fat levels, with insulin diverting glucose into fat cells – as will happen if you consume high-GI foods too regularly and endure 'sugar rushes'.

Given the needs of the training programmes in this book, you should aim for 6–7g of carbohydrate per kg (2lb) of body weight per day. Thus, if you weighed 70kg (154lb) you would need between 420 and 490g (15–17oz) per day. Note: the more lean muscle you gain, the more carbs in the form of glycogen stored in your muscles (and liver) you will need.

Carbohydrate timing and your workouts

It's recommended that you eat something substantial every 2–4 hours and a snack 1–2 hours before training. Experiment with your meal timings to find out what works for you.

In terms of in-workout feeding, water should be sufficient to keep you going as the majority of workouts last less than an hour. Note: becoming dehydrated can significantly impair performance. Try to drink a litre of water for every hour of exercise you do, in addition to that base 2 litres that is constantly recommended. However, it's very important to take an appropriate meal/snack within an hour or so after your workout, to kick-start the recovery and regeneration of your glycogen stores and protein repair.

See the list of suitable post-workout snacks and meals on page 193, which follow the 4 parts carb to 1 part protein ratio deemed optimum for post-workout recovery.

PRE-WORKOUT MEALS

(2–4 hours before exercise)
- Jacket potato with beans, cheese, coleslaw, tuna or chicken
- Pasta with tomato-based sauce, cheese and vegetables
- Chicken with rice and salad
- Porridge with milk
- Fish and potato pie
- Vegetable stir fry with prawns or tofu with noodles or rice

PRE-WORKOUT SNACKS

(1–2 hours before exercise)
- Fresh fruit
- Smoothie
- Yogurt
- Fruit loaf or raisin bread
- Dried apricots, dates and raisins

Source: Adapted from Anita Bean's *The Complete Guide to Sports Nutrition* (6th edition)

SELECTED FOODS CONTAINING 50G/1½oz OF CARBOHYDRATE

- 65g (2¼oz) muesli
- 90g (3oz) oats
- 4 slices of bread (100g/3½oz)
- 2 pittas (100g/3½oz)
- 2 pancakes (150g/5¼oz)
- 180g (6½oz) boiled rice
- 2 medium–large bananas
- 3 medium fruits (e.g. orange, apple)
- 12 small fruits (e.g. apricots)
- 350g (12oz) sweet potato
- 350g (12oz) potato
- 250–300ml (8–10 US fl oz) fruit smoothie

▶ Fat

Fat contains twice as many calories as protein and carbohydrate per gram and our bodies can store it in almost unlimited quantities. Certain types of fat are also harmful to health. These two reasons alone will tell you why we must carefully monitor our fat consumption. Of course, not all fat is bad and we do need some fat, for example, essential fatty acids, to survive. We should stick to obtaining no more than 20–25 per cent of our daily calorific consumption from it. This percentage is below that generally recommended for the main population (30 per cent) and indeed the amount consumed by many people in the Western world is often higher.

Calculations are provided at the end of this section in terms of working out specific fat needs, as this process requires you to do some metabolic rate calculations.

CHOLESTEROL AND FATS

Cholesterol actually performs a number of positive bodily functions. One of these is its assistance in the production of numerous hormones. Although low-density lipoprotein cholesterol is commonly referred to as 'bad', it's only actually bad when its levels in the body are pushed up by factors that include a lack of exercise, obesity and the consumption of too many saturated fats.

TYPES OF FAT
SATURATED FATS

Saturated fats are found mainly, but not exclusively, in dairy and animal products and are traditionally seen as the most 'harmful', as in excess they can raise so-called 'bad' LDL cholesterol and with it the risk of heart disease. It's been recommended for over three decades by the Department of Health in the UK that no more than 10 per cent of daily calories come from this source of fat – however, thoughts on this are now changing and saturated fats are beginning to be seen as less of a potential problem in terms of weight gain and health, as long as a sensible approach to their consumption is followed. Processed and high-sugar carbs and foods are perhaps more of a culprit in terms of weight gain, for example.

The dietary balance advocated in this book emphasizes protein consumption, with carbs and fats being balanced around it. Carbs get a slightly lighter weighting.

UNSATURATED FATS

Monounsaturated fats are found in olive oil, nuts and seeds and can reduce LDL cholesterol and its negative effects. These fats are normally liquid at room temperature. No more than 12 per cent of your daily calories should come from this fat source.

Polyunsaturated fats are found in most vegetable oils, oily fish, nuts and seeds. They are liquid at room temperature and below. No more than 10 per cent of your daily calories should come from this fat source. Note you'll need to pool your consumption of monounsaturated and polyunsaturared fats when assessing your fat consumption as there's a crossover i.e. nuts and seeds contain both monounsaturated and polyunsaturared fats.

Essential Fatty Acids (Omega-3 and Omega-6 series) cannot be produced in the body and must be provided by food – rather like the essential amino acids. Omega-3 essential fatty acids can prevent blood clotting, have anti-inflammatory properties and are beneficial to the immune system.

Omega-3 fats are found in some nuts and seeds, such as flax seeds, walnuts and pumpkin seeds, as well as in soya beans and oily fish, such as sardines, mackerel, salmon, trout, grass fed meats and herrings. Omega-6 fatty acids can reduce LDL (so-called 'bad' cholesterol, see page 198) and are also beneficial for healthy skin, for example. They are found in nuts, seeds, some vegetable oils, such as sunflower, and the germ of whole grains. Specifically in regard to assisting your resistance training, they can:

■ improve oxygen and nutrient transport to cells.

■ improve aerobic energy metabolism.

■ help against strain injuries, as they have anti-inflammatory properties.

■ increase growth hormone secretion as a consequence of sleep and/or exercise.

Aim for 0.9g of Omega-3 a day and 0.2 per cent of total daily calorific requirements from Omega-6.

WHAT IS CHOLESTEROL?

Cholesterol is a part of all cell membranes and is needed by our bodies. It contributes to the production of several hormones. Cholesterol is in part derived from the food we eat, but is in the main produced in the liver from saturated fats. Too much LDL cholesterol is thought to be detrimental to heart health.

TRANS FATS are mainly the result of attempts to prolong the shelf life of monounsaturated and polyunsaturated fats. Some countries have actually banned them/attempted to ban them – so avoid them! Food labels don't currently display trans fat content so to avoid them look for food labels that list hydrogenated or partially hydrogenated oils and vegetable fat instead which are the same thing.

Body fat levels

The rise of technology and access to information, and sometimes a misconstrued – aka media-constructed – appreciation of what the human body should look like has led to many people striving for potentially unrealistic body shapes and body fat levels.

Elite female athletes can achieve minimum levels of body fat of 10 per cent, but this is the extreme. At or around the 10 per cent level, women can suffer from menstrual cycle irregularities (oligomenorrhoea) and cessation (amenorrhoea), infertility and reduced bone density (increasing the risk of stress fractures). Reduced immune system function can also result.

So don't get preoccupied with body fat levels – train and rejoice in the changes that occur to your body naturally as a result of following the 24-week plan and measure your progress in terms of how you feel and move and look. Rather like the scales, only use body fat measurements occasionally and temper your result against more qualitative measures.

More on saturated fat

Saturated fat often gets tarnished as being the bad guy, but it's actually the quantity and type consumed that makes this the case – not, for example, products such as cheese and milk. To reiterate, trans fats are bad and should be avoided. But it's argued that too great a consumption of carbs could actually be of greater concern when it comes to shaping and building a lean body (and, in terms of the bigger picture, reducing obesity levels). Want some evidential proof? Back in 1975, most British people ate 51.7g/approx. 2oz (400 plus calories) of saturated fat a day, this being reduced to 28.1g/approx. 1oz (220 plus calories) by 1999, but obesity rates have sky-rocketed

since then. Obviously other factors such as reduced energy expenditure must be taken into account but it can be seen that perhaps saturated fat is not as much of a problem as it is often thought to be.

Body composition and metabolic rate

In this section, information is provided on metabolic rate. Note that the information will assist you to calculate your daily fat needs, too.

BODY COMPOSITION
Our bodies are composed of different tissue types.

LEAN BODY TISSUE (also known as 'fat free mass') Lean body tissue is made up of muscles, bones, blood and organs. It's metabolically active. As I've stressed,

---

TABLE 12

JUST WHAT DOES REDUCED FAT MEAN?

Label	Fat content
Fat-free	Less than 0.15g of fat per 100g (3½oz)
Low fat	Less than 3g of fat per 100g (3½oz)
Reduced fat	At least 25% less fat than the full fat alternative
Low-fat spread	40g of fat per 100g (3½oz)

The information in the table above is provided for reference – in reality, and in keeping with more recent research on fat (of which more later), it could actually be better to use full-fat products – in moderation, of course.

---

muscle plays a very important role when it comes to fat burning and keeping you lean. It can burn up to three times as many calories as any other part of the body, so basically the leaner you become, the more effective you are as a calorie burning machine. Every 0.45kg/1lb of lean muscle can burn up to 35 calories a day – it doesn't sound much, but multiply that by 365 days a year, every year, and you will begin to see the value.

FAT TISSUE (or adipose tissue)

Fat tissue is made up of:

■ **Essential fat** – this is stored in bone marrow, the heart, lungs and liver and other vital organs and supports life.

■ **Storage fat** – this acts as a sort of cushion that protects the body's vital organs. It's also spread around the body below the skin's surface (as subcutaneous fat).

■ **Non-essential fat** is just that – it has no real purpose and is detrimental to health if you store too much of it.

BODY FAT TESTING

A body fat or body composition test can tell you whether you have too much non-essential fat. The test provides a body fat percentage and some tests also pinpoint where it is distributed. Most gyms/health clubs are able to provide this test. It's also possible to get body fat testing machines for home use. The accuracy of these machines (commercial or otherwise) can vary and may be affected by factors such as your hydration levels. Having said that, they are a much better measure of how your training is progressing compared to weighing scales. This is because lean muscle weighs more than fat – thus it is possible that you could have shaped up, look better and have a much more functional body, despite the scales indicating that you have not lost much weight.

TOTAL DAILY ENERGY EXPENDITURE (TDEE)

Our bodies use energy throughout the day and night to keep us alive – this is known as Total Daily Energy Expenditure (TDEE).

Resting Metabolic Rate (RMR)

A very significant proportion (60–75 per cent) of TDEE is used to maintain Resting Metabolic Rate (RMR). RMR refers to all those unseen and unthought-of essential bodily functions, such as heart, lung and mental functioning. Calculations of RMR are made over a 24-hour period but do not include the calories burned while sleeping (Basal Metabolic Rate refers to the calories burned while asleep).

Activity

The high percentage of calories used to maintain RMR may come as a surprise to many, as it's often assumed that exercise and other physical activity is responsible for the majority of our energy expenditure. However, the reality is that only 15 per cent at most of our TDEE actually goes on any activity. But don't be discouraged by this, as this seemingly small percentage can make a huge difference to any body shaping and fat loss goals and the creation of a positive energy balance. And as noted, in the case of resistance training it can build a very extensive fat burning machine – aka you!

Thermic Effect of Feeding (TEF)

The Thermic Effect of Feeding (TEF) makes up the remaining 10 per cent of daily energy expenditure. When food is consumed, energy is burned. This in part explains why eating five to six times throughout the day can have a better effect on fat burning and balancing blood sugar levels than eating bigger meals less frequently. And it also explains why we warm up after we eat.

🏋 How to...

The following steps show you how to calculate your metabolic rate and your daily calorific requirements (including training and activity level) and express this as a specific macronutrient split.

▶ Step 1: Estimate your RMR

The information (right) will enable you to calculate your metabolic rate while following the plans in this book.

CALCULATE METABOLIC RATE

Age	Formula	Results for 70kg (154lb) person in kcal
10–18	Body weight in kg x 12.2 + 746	1,600
19–30	Body weight in kg x 14.7 + 496	1,525
31–60	Body weight in kg x 8.7+ 829	1,438

▶ Step 3: Add workout calories
FITNESS ACTIVITIES AND CALORIE BURNING

Information on the calorie burning potential of selected fitness and resistance training options per hour and per minute is provided to the right. You'll see that the 'burn' from weight training is not insignificant. The higher figure would most likely result from short recovery workouts, involving lots of compound moves, such as the Legs, Bottom and Core, Lower Body Metabolic Blaster and All Body Workout Blast found in the first 12 weeks of the training programme (Chapter 4) and the Kettlebell Dominant All-body Workout found in Chapter 5. Pyramid workouts and those with low reps and longer recoveries are more likely to burn calories at the lower end of the scale.

FITNESS ACTIVITIES AND CALORIE BURNING

Activity	Kcal/hour	Approx. Kcal/min
Weight training	270–450	4.5–7.5
Aerobics (high intensity)	520	8.5
Boxing (sparring)	865	14
Cycling (16 km/hour)	384	6.4
Cycling (8.8 km/hour)	250	4.2
Rowing (moderate)	445	7.4
Swimming (fast)	630	10.5
Swimming (for fitness)	615	10.2
Treadmill running (5.6 min/km)	750	12.5
Treadmill running (3.8 min/km)	1,000	16.6

The above figures are based on a 70kg (154lb) individual. If you weigh more you'll burn more calories, if less you'll burn fewer calories. Your fitness level will also play a key determining role – in general, the fitter you are the fewer calories you'll burn.

Step 2: Factor in your daily (non-workout) level

MULTIPLE FOR LEVEL OF ACTIVITY

Daily level of activity	Defined per day by...	Multiple	Total calorific needs for 70kg (154lb person)
Mostly sedentary	Standing or seated most of the day	1.4	2,240
Moderately active	Regular brisk walks or similar	1.7	2,592
Very active	Regular physical activity	2.0	2,876

To estimate your resistance/weight training workout needs:

Calorific needs for 70kg (154lb) person (RMR + activity level multiple)	Total daily requirement plus added weight training calories (estimated on 4 workouts a week at 300 kcal/hour average)
2,240	2,540
2,592	2,892
2,876	3,176

Step 4: Calculate your fat needs

At the beginning of this chapter, information on your protein and carb needs was provided, based on grams of the macronutrients per kg (2lb) of body weight. It's recommended that fat calories be calculated on the basis of protein and carb needs. To recap on protein and carbs:

■ **Protein:** If you weigh 70kg (154lb), you need to consume between 112g and 133g/4-5oz) of protein per day (1.6–1.9g/approx.½oz of protein per day per kg/2lb of body weight). This equates to 448–532 kcal, as there are 4 kcal in 1g of protein.

■ **Carbohydrate:** If you weigh 70kg (154lb), you need to consume between 420g and 490g (15–17oz of carbohydrate per day (6–7g/ approx. ¼oz of carbohydrate per kg/2lb of body weight per day). This equates to 1,680–1,960 kcal as there are 4 kcal in 1g of carbohydrate.

■ **Fat:** Your daily fat calories would be determined by subtracting the number of carbohydrate + protein calories from your estimated daily metabolic needs. So a very active 70kg (154lb) woman would need around 3,176 calories on a workout day, of which 532 would come from protein and 1,960 from carbs (calculated at upper range). These two figures added together are 2,492; subtract this from your workout day's estimated calorie needs to leave 684 fat calories. As there are 9kcal in 1 fat gram, this equates to about 76g (2¼oz) of fat.

SUMMARY OF CALORIFIC NEEDS FOR A 70KG (154LB) WOMAN ON A RESISTANCE TRAINING DAY:

Protein	133g x 4 kcal/g	=	532 kcal
Carbs	490g x 4 kcal/g	=	1,960 kcal
Fat	76g x 9 kcal/g	=	684 kcal
	Total	=	3,176 kcal

▶ Factors to consider when making your calculations

■ The figures for the workout calorie consumption have been estimated and averaged out at the top end of the scale and you will need to make more specific day-to-day calculations. Using an app (and your smartphone) or a heart rate monitor with a calorie burning function could assist in calculating a more exact number of calories expended by specific workouts. However, as with body fat monitors and heart rate monitor functions, these apps can be inaccurate.

■ You need to be mindful of the fact that you need to consume fewer calories on the days when you are not working out (to calculate your daily requirement here, simply deduct calories that would have been expended for exercise).

■ It's important to be aware that regular training will increase your metabolic rate on a day-to-day basis by as much as 17 per cent due to excess post-workout oxygen consumption.

Tip: keep your heart rate monitor on after training to gain an indication of the increased calorie burn post workout.

■ Finally, there's the boost to metabolic rate that being leaner can give – lean muscle burns more calories.

So there are many factors to consider when trying to be exact in calculating your calorie needs.

NEED YOUR BODY FAT MEASUREMENT AND RMR TO BE EXACT?

At £40/$61 (at the time of writing) for an exact and accessible body fat reading, the BodPod offers great potential and a starting point for those of you who are serious about ensuring your training and eating habits remain fully and accurately on track. The BodPod is an egg-like chamber that uses air displacement to measure body fat levels.

BodPod providers (and others) can also test your RMR – the test measures the oxygen and carbon dioxide content of your breath over a 45-minute resting period while you are hooked up to the test kit. This test, too, will provide very accurate results.

Both tests are available from the British College of Osteopathic Medicine (www.bcom.ac.uk). Or you can locate a relevant site at: http://www.bodpod.com

▶ Resistance training dietary tip: Don't yo-yo diet.

Restricting your calories by going on a crash diet can lead to short-term weight loss but long-term weight gain. Our bodies are designed to hang on to calories when food is scarce – this is a legacy from our prehistoric ancestors' days. It will attempt to eke out as much energy as possible from every gram of food it consumes if it thinks that more food will be a long time coming. Yo-yo diets therefore slow your metabolic rate and stunt fat burning/weight loss. Additionally it's probable you won't get the nutrients (macro and micro) that you need to optimally meet your body's requirements and support your resistance training

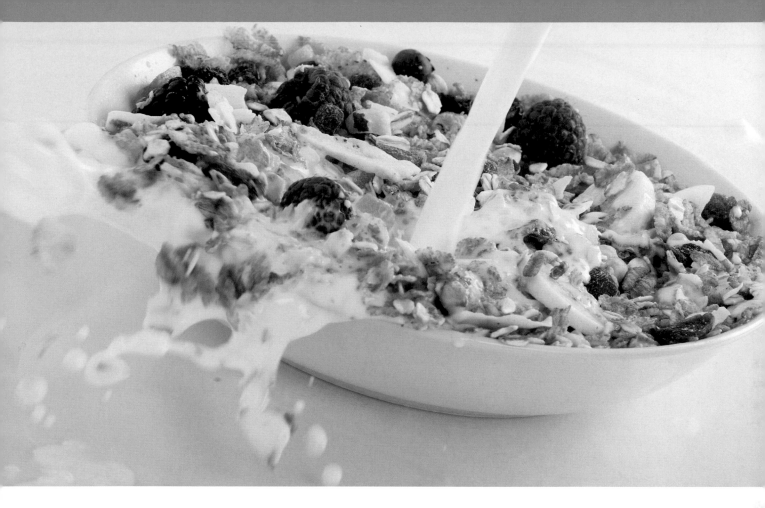

efforts. So don't yo-yo diet and extensively cut calories if weight loss is your goal. Eat according to your activity and workout needs, using the advice provided. As a guide, don't under-eat (or overeat for that matter, if weight gain is your aim) by more than 15 per cent of total daily calorie consumption.

▶ What to eat on a resistance training day

Here you'll find an idea of what you could typically eat on a resistance training day. Coupled with the information on how to calculate your macronutrient needs, you'll be in a great position to get your resistance training nutrition right.

BREAKFAST

Breakfast really is the most important meal of the day. If you don't consume sufficient calories first thing, you'll run the risk of not having enough energy to get you through the day – or, more likely, to mid-morning. A high carbohydrate, low-fat start is what's required – this will enhance both mental and physical mood and get energy levels up. You need carbs that will both kick-start and drip energy for the next few hours.

Grab a bowl of muesli – it'll provide 33g of carbohydrate energy – and use semi-skimmed milk, which contains only 2.8 per cent of fat per 100g. Eat some fruit for a great energy source. Fruits with a low GI, such as plums and oranges, will release their energy slowly over the next few hours. To maintain energy levels, bagels are another great breakfast option – high in carbohydrates and low in fat, you could combine them with honey or peanut butter.

MID-MORNING

If you feel peckish around 11am, an energy bar makes a good choice. It'll provide around 150 low-fat, high-carbohydrate calories. Raisin scones make another good choice.

LUNCH

A pasta-based meal will set you up nicely for an early evening workout. Pasta releases its energy slowly over a period of two to four hours. A 100g/1 cup (raw weight) portion will provide 76 grams of carbohydrate.

MID-AFTERNOON

A similar snack to the one you had mid-morning should keep you going nicely.

A banana, a handful of raisins or an energy bar will provide a further quick energy release if needed before your workout.

WORKOUT

If your workout lasts more than an hour, then consuming additional carbohydrate can improve your performance. To derive maximum benefit, it's crucial that this process is started within the first half an hour of the workout and you should aim for 30–60g of carbohydrate. This 'in-workout refuelling' should enable you to exercise for at least a further 45 minutes relatively comfortably. However, as noted, the majority of your workouts should last only an hour so this will probably not be needed. The information is useful for reference.

POST WORKOUT

As we have seen, the first hour or two after your workout is the optimum time to eat and rehydrate to maximise your body's recovery processes and maximise gains. Exercise burns glycogen and breaks down muscle protein – eating the right foods and in the right quantities post workout will significantly kick-start recovery and refuel for the next workout. It'll also have the added benefit of keeping your metabolism nicely ticking over and avoid sugar crashes.

After a workout, aim for at least 2g of carbohydrate per kg of body weight and 40g of protein. That's 140g (4.9oz) of carbohydrate for a 70kg (154lb) person.

500ml (17 US fl oz) of diluted fruit juice will provide 30g (1oz) of carbohydrate, as will 500ml of an isotonic sports drink.

More examples of suitable post-workout snacks:
- Dried fruit
- Bread roll with honey
- Flavoured milk

EVENING MEAL

You could go for a jacket potato filled with beans, fish, chicken or cheese. Lean beef, chicken and preferably brown rice are also great choices – they'll continue the refuelling and recovery process and keep your energy levels elevated.

PRE-SLEEP

On tough resistance training days, a protein source prior to sleep could assist protein regrowth and recovery overnight. Casein is a slow release protein – a good source is cheese. Cottage cheese is often recommended as a suitable pre-bed protein snack. A suitable casein protein supplement would also be a suitable alternative.

HYDRATION

Drinking two litres of water a day will prevent dehydration and keep your energy levels up throughout the day. However, on workout days aim to increase your fluid consumption by an additional 0.5 to 1 litre for every hour of exercise you do. You'll know if you are properly hydrated as your urine will be clear and odourless.

Dehydration can significantly affect your workout performance
A 3–5 per cent loss in body weight caused by dehydration can significantly impair judgement, mental sharpness and reaction time as well as aerobic performance. A runner could lose 1.2 litres of water running at 6-minute-mile pace on a cool 10°C day and a loss of just 2 per cent (that's 2.0kg/4.4lb if you weigh 70kg/154lb) in body weight caused by dehydration could impair performance by 10–20 per cent. Note: although this tends to affect aerobic exercises more than anaerobic resistance trainers, you can't neglect your hydration if you want to make maximal progress. Water is crucial to all body processes.

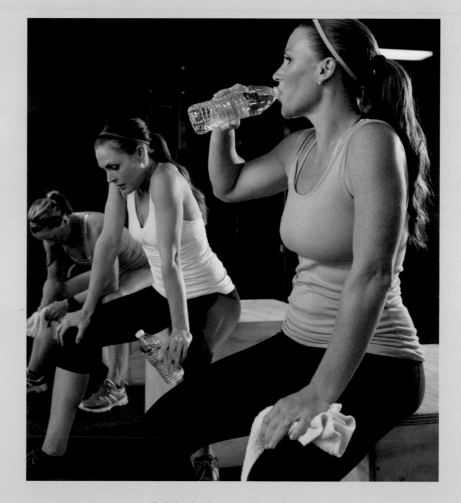

Drink alcohol moderately
Alcohol has no nutritional value and is high in calories (7 per calorie). A glass of red wine contains 85 kcal and a shot of vodka, whisky or gin contains 55 kcal. It's a hot topic right now, due to its potential contribution to high obesity levels, with calls for the calorific content of alcohol to be made available on labels and in bars and clubs.

Micronutrients

▶ Minerals and vitamins

Minerals and vitamins are your body's spark plugs. They perform a myriad of vital functions, enhance vitality and can optimise your workouts.

MINERALS

Twenty-two mainly metallic minerals make up 4 per cent of body mass. Their main function is to balance and regulate internal chemistry – for example, they play a crucial role in the maintenance of muscle contractions, regulation of heartbeat and nerve conduction.

▼ Aim to eat a rainbow of fruit and vegetables each day.

VITAMINS

Vitamins are vital, for example, in terms of maximising energy release from food and aiding recovery from workouts and injuries, but do not produce energy themselves. As with minerals, consuming excess amounts (above the recommended Reference Nutrient Intake/Recommended Daily Allowance) does not enhance their metabolic contribution.

Table 13 breaks down what selected vitamins and minerals can do for you from the perspective of enhancing fitness – obviously they have many other positive health benefits too. Table 14 indicates how much valuable micronutrient content can be lost when selected foods are processed. The moral here: don't buy processed foods.

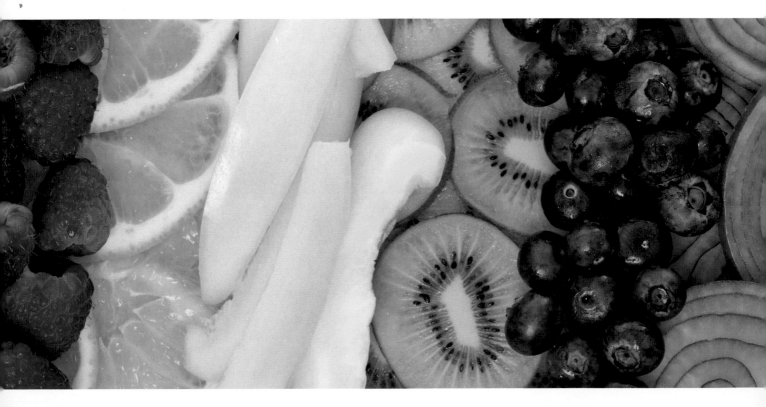

REFERENCE NUTRIENT INTAKE (RNI) OF SELECTED VITAMINS AND MINERALS

Antioxidant vitamins and minerals	Reference Nutrient Intake (RNI) per day	Sources
A (vitamin)	600mcg	Dairy products, oily fish, liver, butter
Beta-carotene (vitamin)	15–25mg (suggested intake – no official RNI)	Bright red, green, orange and yellow vegetables
C (vitamin)	60mg	Citrus and other fresh fruits, vegetables (particularly dark green leafy ones), berries
E (vitamin)	No official UK RNI EU recommendation – 10mg	Pure vegetable oils, nuts, sunflower seeds, avocado, wholemeal bread
Selenium (mineral)	60mcg	Tuna, oysters, herrings, cottage cheese, seafood

• RNI is the measure used in the UK. RDA (Recommended Daily Allowance) is the measure preferred by the European Union.

• The amounts shown are guidelines only – no two people's needs will be the same. Variation will result according to gender, age and training levels, for example.

TABLE 13

UNDERSTANDING UNITS OF MEASUREMENT

You'll be familiar with the unit of weight called a gram – it's about the weight of a Smartie. Apart from calcium and potassium, the amounts of each nutrient required by the body each day are much less than a gram so other, much smaller units are used.

■ **The milligram** is abbreviated mg and is one thousandth of a gram. There are 1,000mgs in a gram.

■ **The microgram** is abbreviated mcg and is one millionth of a gram. There are 1,000mcgs in each milligram.

■ **The International Unit** is abbreviated I.U. It's sometimes used instead of mgs or mcgs for vitamins such as A, D and E where there is more than one form of a vitamin. International units express the biological activity that different forms of vitamins exhibit.

FOOD PROCESSING, MINERAL LOSS IN SELECTED STAPLE FOODS

	White flour	Refined Sugar	White rice
Chromium	98%	95%	92%
Zinc	78%	88%	54%
Manganese	86%	89%	75%

TABLE 14

Antioxidants and phytochemicals

A diet rich in antioxidants (vitamins A, C, E and beta-carotene and the mineral selenium) and phytochemicals will prevent free radical damage to cells, reduce so-called 'bad' LDL cholesterol and defend our bodies against age-related diseases such as heart disease and cancer. These vitamins and minerals are especially important when you are in hard training. Tough workouts can increase free radical cell damage. What does this mean? Well, we need oxygen to survive – it fuels our heart and lungs and all other bodily processes, including energy release from food. Unfortunately, oxygen metabolism can create unstable molecular fragments, which can damage our cells if left unchecked. It's also been found that the muscular soreness that occurs after tough resistance training can increase the circulation of free radicals. Antioxidant vitamins, minerals and phytochemicals help combat this cellular damage.

PHYTOCHEMICALS

We don't need phytochemicals to survive, so they are not regarded as nutrients, but they do play a vital role in maintaining health. There are over 100 phytochemicals and, like essential amino acids (see page 193), they cannot be stored in the body – examples include bioflavonoids, phytoestrogens, capsaicin and allium compounds. Table 15 summarises selected phytochemical sources and their positive health benefits.

To ensure a plentiful supply of antioxidants and phytochemicals in our diet, we need to eat a variety of plant foods, rice, bread, pasta and seven to eight daily servings of fruit and vegetables. This can include fruit juice and 'smoothies'. Many supermarkets now display the 'daily serving' of a particular fruit and vegetable source – you'll soon realise that you don't need to leave the supermarket with a wheelbarrow full of fruit and vegetables to consume the required amount.

POSITIVE HEALTH BENEFITS OF SELECTED PHYTOCHEMICALS

Phytochemical	Source	Health benefit
Allium compounds	Onions, garlic, chives, shallots	Can combat cancer and benefit the immune system
Bioflavonoids	Rosehips, citrus fruits, berries, grapes, tea, red wine	Antioxidant Can act as an antibiotic and benefit bleeding gums, bruises and soft tissue injuries
Ellagic acid	Strawberries, grapes and raspberries	Can combat cancer
Phytoestrogens	Soya, tofu, citrus fruits, pulses, wheat and celery	Significant effect on reducing the onset of breast and prostate cancer and can reduce the hormonal responses associated with the menopause

TABLE 15

How to get the most out of your resistance and CV workouts with minerals and vitamins

The vitamins and minerals listed in Table 16 have been selected for their ability to enhance your workouts.

SPECIFIC WORKOUT-ENHANCING MINERALS AND VITAMINS

Vitamin/mineral	Function	Reference Nutrient Intake (RNI) per day	Sources
Biotin (vitamin)	Assists glycogen manufacture and protein metabolism for muscle building	No UK RNI – 0.1–0.2mg is recommended	Egg yolk, nuts, oats, whole grains
Calcium (mineral)	Assists muscle contraction	700mg	Dairy products, seafood, vegetables, bread, pulses
Iron (mineral)	Can assist CV exercise	14.8mg	Liver, red meat, pasta, cereals, green leafy vegetables
Zinc (mineral)	Important for metabolising proteins, carbohydrates and fats	7mg	Lean meat and fish, eggs, wholegrain cereals, dairy products
Magnesium (mineral)	Boosts energy production and assists muscle contraction, appears to play a role in blood sugar stabilisation	270mg	Green leafy vegetables, fruit, unrefined whole grains and cereals

TABLE 16

EAT TO BOOST RECOVERY

Nutrition to reduce soft-tissue and cellular (free radical) damage

Vitamin C
Vitamin C plays a crucial role in the formation of collagen. Collagen is a protein that forms the basis for connective tissue (muscles, ligaments and tendons). Specifically, vitamin C acts as a catalyst that stimulates other body chemicals to construct collagen. Vitamin C is also an antioxidant.

Source of vitamin C: citrus fruits, green peppers, leafy dark green vegetables and strawberries.

Bioflavonoids
Bioflavonoids also play an anti-inflammatory role (inflammation is behind diseases such as heart disease and cancer). They are found in brightly coloured fruits and vegetables and are part of the group of nutrients called phytochemicals (see page 210). Bioflavonoids are also antioxidants.

JOINT PAIN – THE POTENTIALITY OF GLUCOSAMINE SULPHATE AND CHONDROITIN SUPPLEMENTATION

Research indicates that use of the supplements glucosamine sulphate and chondroitin can potentially reduce joint damage such as osteoarthritis.

Glucosamine is used in the manufacture of very large molecules found in joint cartilage. Basically, these hold on to water, rather like a sponge, and it's thought that, in doing so, they provide cushioning for joints. Research indicates that chondroitin heads straight to the joints and lumbar discs when it is ingested. Surveys also indicate that, although more limited in extent when compared with glucosamine, chondroitin reduces pain and increases mobility.

To build up working levels of glucosamine and chondroitin in the body, try a combined supplement, ingesting 1,500mg daily.

Cod liver oil
Along the same lines, cod liver oil can also reduce inflammation and contribute to joint health. The key ingredient is the essential fatty acid Omega-3. Eating oily fish regularly (once or twice a week) will reduce the need to use supplements.

Brooke Stacey

MODEL OF RESISTANCE-TRAINED FITNESS

'About four years ago, I transformed my body and reassessed my health and fitness goals. After I graduated from college and began working full time in sales I found myself wanting to lose weight – specifically the 4.5kg/10lbs that I couldn't seem to get off. I hired a personal trainer and went to work. I never anticipated what the end result would be, but after six months of training I ended up with a transformed body that I had not thought was possible. As a result I got some modelling work with fitness magazines and decided to qualify as a personal trainer. I wanted to be able to better educate myself and others on my new-found passion for health and fitness.

'My training from week-to-week can vary depending on the programme my trainer has me on and the goals we are trying to achieve such as building more muscle or leaning up, while maintaining the muscle I currently have. We try to switch up my training routine every month to ensure my body continues to be challenged and is changing toward reaching my current goal. My workouts are set around my work scheduling. For this reason, intensity in my workouts is crucial to the success of my body responding – we can't always get to the gym five

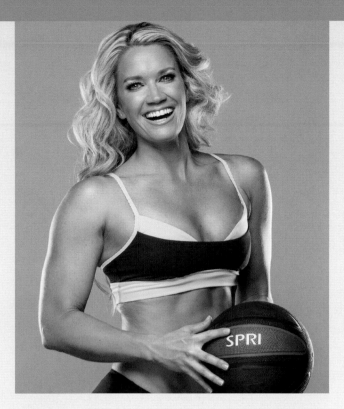

days a week. This is also the beauty of a great workout programme – it can provide some variability and still be successful. Consistency in clean eating helps me stay on track with achieving my goals in the gym no matter if I'm lifting three or five days a week.

'My favourite exercises are always with free weights. I enjoy lifting heavy and engaging my entire body during my lifting ... so for me it's standing shoulder press and dumbbell chest press because I am strongest in my shoulders and chest and I love the adrenaline rush I get from lifting heavy! My least favourite exercises are biceps curls and sit-ups.

▶ Advice

'My advice to anyone wanting to get as fit as they can is to get started, keep going and never limit yourself to what is possible. The body is an incredible thing and can achieve

beyond what your mind would otherwise limit it to. If you consistently train and eat healthily, the end results are limitless. Transformations are possible and happen every day. It's a matter of how important it is to you and what work you are willing to do to see the results.

▶ Diet

'I truly don't follow a diet. I focus on eating clean all the time. When I transformed my body I slowly began to make changes to my eating habits like cutting back on fast food, limiting fried foods, incorporating more vegetables and taking out processed snack foods like chips, crackers and cookies. I avoid processed foods and try to eat natural, organic foods as much as possible. I have never been on a diet for a show or shoot. I eat the same all-year round and adjust my workouts and clean up my eating when I get closer to a shoot date. By applying a holistic approach to eating I find it is easy to follow and maintain my clean eating and I don't feel like I have to deprive myself.

'My tip for anyone trying to eat better and avoid cravings is to look at the whole picture when preparing a meal or eating out. Try to make every meal as healthy as you can, like baking instead of frying and use lean meats and veggies instead of white starches. This approach has worked for me from the beginning and makes it a lifestyle I can maintain long-term versus a diet that comes and goes. When you don't deprive yourself or go on strict diets you will be less likely to crave and binge-eat foods that will sabotage your health and fitness goals.'

To find out more about Brooke search for Brooke Stacey Fitness Model on Facebook.

🏋 Supplements

If you believe some of the hype from supplement manufacturers (and purveyors of diet foods), after one swig of, for example, a protein shake, you'd be super-fit, super-slim, have optimum lean muscle mass levels and be the embodiment of health and vitality! Oh, if only it were so simple. The answer to whether you should use supplements or not is, as I've said before, in their name – they are supplements. This means that they are supplemental to your optimised real food consumption. The information provided in this chapter will enable you to construct and follow such a diet.

▶ Do they work?

The other point for consideration is – do they work? Obviously, the supplement manufacturers will claim they do. The reality is that some are much more beneficial than others and some are redundant provided you follow a healthy diet. A case in point in terms of the latter are protein supplements – if you follow the recommendations in this chapter in terms of macronutrient selection, then it's very unlikely that you will need to supplement with additional protein (of course, lifestyle considerations may have an influence – supplements can be useful if you don't have time to prepare/eat real food). Having said that, there are some supplements that have proven (or at least more proven) results and are potentially very useful for resistance training – of which more later. And if you use these and carefully consider the use of others (in terms of when you are eating on the run, for example, and don't have time to properly prepare your food), then supplements can have a role to play in terms of getting the most from your training and everyday health and fitness.

▶ Creatine

Creatine is one of the most well-known of all sports supplements. It's naturally produced in the body by the liver and kidneys (from three amino acids). It's found in muscles, where it is used to produce energy. Research indicates that loading muscles with additional creatine through supplementation will increase your exercise potential. This means, for example, that you'll be able to perform more repetitions and sets when weight training or when performing similar short-lasting anaerobic energy-

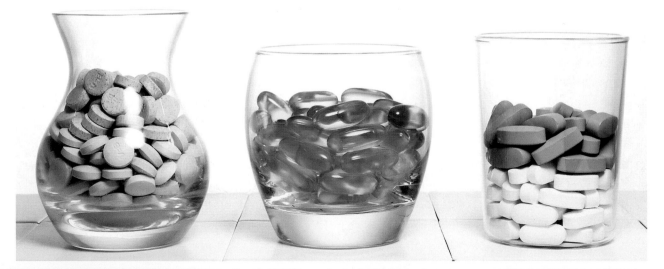

based activities, such as sprinting.

Regular creatine supplementation can increase lean muscle by an average of 2.5kg (5½lb), which also makes it a great fat burning supplement – the leaner your muscle mass, the better a fat burner your body will be.

Any 'downsides' are more anecdotal than proven. Some people experience greater levels of muscular cramping when taking creatine, so to avoid this you should increase your fluid intake.

Creatine can be purchased in different forms, but it's probably best to get it as pure creatine monohydrate powder and mix this with fruit juice.

Creatine requires a loading dose (normally 4 x 5g a day for 5 days) and then a maintenance dose of 2g a day thereafter (read and follow the manufacturer's recommendations). Note that once you have followed the loading and subsequent maintenance dose for about a month, no further benefit will be gained, so stop using it, come off it for another month and then commence another cycle.

Creatine is naturally found in herring, beef, tuna, pork, salmon, milk and prawns. Note: diet alone could not creatine-load to the extent that supplementation can, although it could make a significant contribution to the usually recommended 2g/day amount.

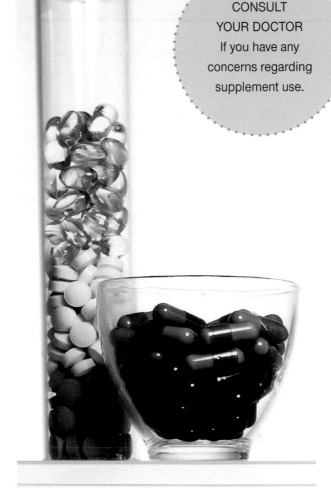

CONSULT YOUR DOCTOR If you have any concerns regarding supplement use.

▶ Glutamine

Glutamine is found in muscle cells and is made from three amino acids. It's essential for cell growth and immune system function.

Positive benefits: glutamine can boost muscle recovery after periods of heavy training.

Supplement recommendation: 2–3g/day.

▶ HMB (beta-hydroxy beta methylbutyrate)

Positive benefits: HMB can increase muscle mass and reduce body fat, probably because it's involved in cellular repair, and also reduce muscle damage.

Supplement recommendation: 2g/day.

8 STAYING ON COURSE

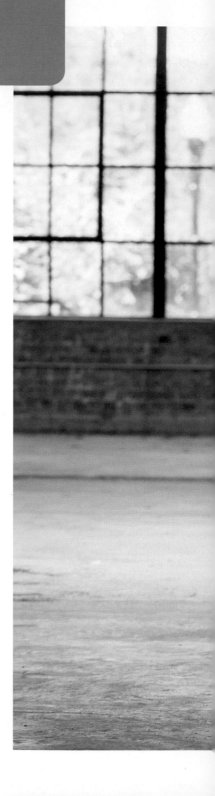

We all lose motivation from time to time but those people who are successful in whatever they seek to achieve are those who generally stick with it and keep motivated. It is perseverance and determination that counts. When it comes to getting fit and fitter, once you know what to do and what to eat (in short, what's in this book!), then it's mostly just a case of repetition to get the results. But staying motivated for the course can prove difficult – there are so many distractions in our lives and we are so time-poor that our workouts, for example, can easily be moved to another day that may never happen. We may also become frustrated and possess unrealistic beliefs about what we can achieve, or we may possess negative traits that have to be challenged if we are going to enjoy and appreciate what we are striving for. This chapter is designed to provide you with some strategies, tips and thoughts that will keep you positive and enable you to stay the resistance training and nutrition course.

1 REACQUAINT YOURSELF WITH THE ROLE MODELS IN THIS BOOK

Firstly, reacquaint yourself with the personal stories of the women who have appeared on the pages of this book. For example, Anita Coleman, Sonjia Ashby, and Emily Lingard – they've all worked out how to make resistance training a central part of their well-being and they are all women no doubt living similar lives to the one you are leading. Their stories emphasise why resistance training is so important, for shaping a great body and as a way to feel good and vital and confident in and about yourself. In many ways, their stories should be the only boost you need... but just to help you that bit more, here are a few other tips and strategies you can use.

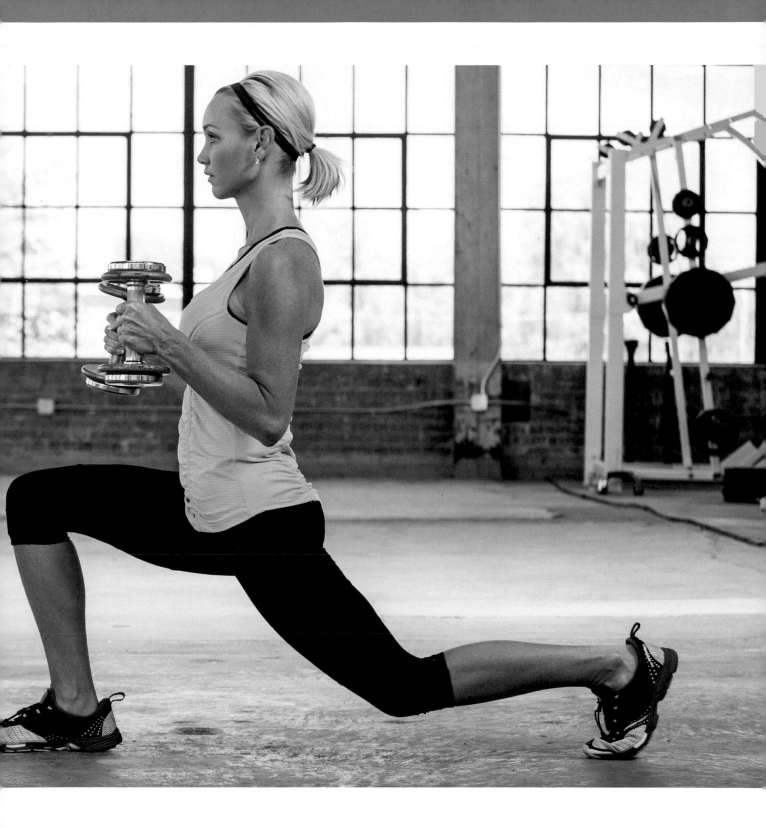

2 USE SOCIAL MEDIA

Today there are groups for virtually everything on social media sites, such as Twitter, Instagram, Pinterest and Facebook.

Anita Coleman, for example, has thousands of followers on her Instagram accounts – one of her pages is aptly called '@mumsthatlift'. Anita acts as a role model and also posts numerous easy to prepare recipes, which you could incorporate into your busy schedule.

Talking to people who share the same belief in working out and lifting weights will make it so much easier for you to follow your lifestyle choices and not be distracted by those who erroneously think that weights and resistance training are not for women and, worse still, that being fit is not worthwhile. Don't succumb to the people who 'can't be bothered' – those who can be described as 'energy vampires', of which more later.

So search social media, sign up now and make contact and talk with, and be inspired by, these like-minded people.

3 BE SURROUNDED BY THE 'RIGHT' PEOPLE

You can do this virtually and – just as importantly, if not more so – in person. You need friends who support what you do and not those who try to dissuade you and suck out your passion. I've heard these people described as 'energy vampires'. You probably know someone like this – we all have them in our circles. Well, now could be the time to show them the garlic or silver dagger if they continue to drain you and take you away from what you really want – your dreams and goals. You should have people around you who realistically support and challenge you, not those who don't respect what you want to do and try to pull you off your chosen, tempered and realistic path.

4 BE REALISTIC – BODY IMAGE

It takes time to make the changes you want, so be patient. At least the information in this book will provide you with the best possible chance of making any body shaping/image dreams you have a reality. However, be realistic when it comes to your body image and your self-perception. Train to your type and shape and optimise you. Don't strive to attain a body that the media creates – most of the time these are so unrealistic and far from healthy as well. So focus on your achievements, i.e. all the workouts you have done and the changes you have made and are making. Rejoice, pat yourself on the back and take confidence.

5 TAKE BABY STEPS

If you look too far ahead, then the journey to travel may appear too long. You may think that training for 24 weeks, 4–5 times a week is a long time, too long perhaps, however, if you take it one week at a time you will soon be able to look back and see where you have travelled from. It's all about those baby steps.

6 DON'T COMPARE – LOOK TO *YOU*

Write it all down, take pictures, set up your own social media page and tell the world what you are doing to make positive change.

This recommendation follows on from those above. Yes, we all tend to look sideways and wish that we had what someone else has – whether this be their lifestyle, money, looks or body and so on. The chances are, however, that these people will also be looking and striving for qualities and achievements that belong to someone else. You'll have heard it many times before when reading motivational texts and articles but it really *is* important to aim to be the best *you* can be and to rejoice in *your* achievements and *your* journey. Doing this will bolster your

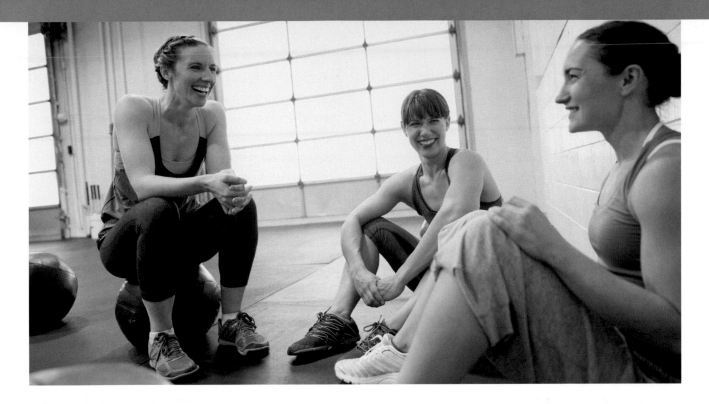

self-esteem and reduce feelings of unhappiness and those that can manifest themselves into feelings of not being good enough. If you look to *you – you'll* feel stronger, more positive and more confident. Really value what you have achieved and are achieving and – in the context of this book – the changes you are making by following the workout and nutritional programmes provided. Write it all down, take pictures, set up your own social media page and tell the world what you are doing to make positive change. You might think you are being egotistical, but if you temper your comments and your progress with the realism of your journey (the good and the bad) and the progress you make day to day, you *will* be an inspiration.

7 ACCEPT THERE WILL BE BAD DAYS

You'll have days when a workout or your nutrition does not go to plan. Accept it and move on. Don't beat yourself up by focusing on what didn't happen. You've another day tomorrow to get back on track. We all have days when we

don't achieve what we were aiming for, but this should not be allowed to bring everything else tumbling down. When it comes to resistance training, once you have got to a certain point, it becomes relatively easy to catch back up, providing your training is/has been relatively consistent. You'll develop what's called 'muscle memory' and you'll be surprised by just how quickly your mind and body respond. Now, I'm not recommending that you start the programme, do three weeks and then take a month off – rather, I'm saying that a day's workout missed here and there won't be a problem. And after completing the 24-week programme, you'll find it will be a lot easier to maintain the fitness and strength and body shape you have attained.

8 VISUALISATION AND MEDITATION

There are numerous ways that you can train your mind to improve your workout, exercise adherence, nutrition commitment and confidence. Visualization can really put you into that place where you want to be. You can see yourself fit and strong and confident; you can see yourself in the gym looking great and enjoying your workouts; you can see yourself in your workout gear, confident in your body... the list goes on. The power of thought cannot and must not be overlooked. When visualizing, the brain can't make out what's real and what's not. If you see yourself lifting strongly and powerfully and training hard, then the chances are you will feel it and actually do it. Finding 10–15 minutes a day to sit and visualise and meditate can significantly improve the physical aspects of your workouts and your approach and attitude towards them, as well as many other aspects of your life and your general wellbeing.

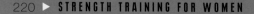

TRY THIS NOW:

- Sit back and relax in a quiet environment, close your eyes and breathe slowly, relaxing all your muscles.
- See yourself in the shape that you want to be.
- You can be training in the gym – anywhere in the world, for that matter. Want to feel the sun on your back while you work out? Then put yourself in that environment!
- Go through one of the workouts in this book in your mind. You will lift every weight you attempt (you can't fail in your mind's eye).
- Feel yourself confident and strong.
- Congratulate yourself and come up with a mantra that you can repeat in your mind when you are in need, for example, of a workout boost. An example: 'I'm fit, strong and have a body that can lift strongly. I am getting fitter and fitter and am in control.'

If you do this regularly and use different visualizations and meditations, you can do much to remove self-doubt and limit negative subconscious thoughts that appear more often than we would like. There are personal trainers and of course councellors who are qualified in Neuro-Linguistic Programming, for example, and they can be of great use in adding that something extra to your well-being in the gym and away from it.

Your journey starts and ends with you. You now have the tools – the training plans, the nutrition tips and the whys and hows – so now it's over to you to train consistently, focused, determined and confident that you will achieve. Oh, and enjoy yourself!

REFERENCES

1 J Strength Cond Res. 2014 Apr 14. [Epub ahead of print]

2 J Strength Cond Res. 2013 Oct; 27(10):2879–86. doi: 10.1519/JSC.0b013e318280d4e2.

3 J Am Geriatr Soc. 1993 Mar; 41(3):205–10.

4 J Appl Physiol (1985). 1995 Sep; 79(3):818–23.

5 Med Sci Sports Exerc. 2001; 33(6):932–8

6 Sports Med. 1991 Feb; 11(2):78–101

7 Br J Sports Med. 1990; 24(2):95–8

8 Sports Med. 2002; 32(15):987–1004

9 Eur J Appl Physiol Occup Physiol. 1993;66(3):254–62.

10 J Strength Cond Res. 2014 May 2

11 J Sci Med Sport. 2014 Jan 30

12 Med Sport Sci. 2012;59:94–103. doi: 10.1159/000341968. Epub 2012 Oct 15

13 J Am Coll Nutr. 2005 Dec;24(6 Suppl):537S–46S

14 Eur J Sport Sci. 2014 Jul 11:1–8. [Epub ahead of print]

15 Eur J Sport Sci. 2014 Jul 11:1–8. [Epub ahead of print]

INDEX

Index entries in *italic* are specific exercises